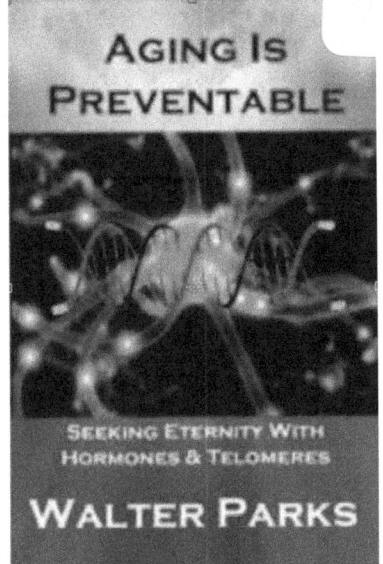

AGING IS PREVENTABLE

SEEKING ETERNITY WITH HORMONES & TELOMERES

WALTER PARKS

Aging is Preventable

By Walter Parks

UnKnownTruths

Publishing Company

8815 Conroy Windermere Rd. Ste 190

Orlando, FL 32835

info@UnknownTruthBooks.com

Contents

Introduction

"Over half the baby boomers here in America are going to see their hundredth birthday and beyond in excellent health. We're looking at life spans for the baby boomers and the generation after the baby boomers of 120 to 150 years of age." Dr. Ronald Klatz, American Academy Of Anti-Aging

"The overall deterioration of the body that comes with growing old is not inevitable." Dr. Rudman, After His Experiments

We can slow, cure, or prevent almost all aging effects if we catch the age-causing problem soon enough. Aging Is Preventable.

I had several TIAs (mini-strokes) seventeen years ago and lost my memory. My doctors fixed my problem with stents and drugs. I have my memory back, and today it is perfect.

I had a heart attack sixteen years ago and another ten years ago. My doctors fixed my problem with stents and drugs. I have had no problems for these last ten years.

I had prostate cancer and got focused radiation six years ago. I have been completely cured. My PSA tests have been very low for these last six years.

I had cataracts in both eyes and underwent surgery. I now see perfectly.

I developed glaucoma, which increases pressure in the eyes and can lead to severe vision problems. I have been taking medicated eye drops for four years, and my eye pressure has returned to normal. I suffer no adverse consequences; except I will have to take the eye drops for the rest of my life.

I developed diabetes three years ago, but I caught it early enough to prevent its progression. I was able to take medications to control my glucose levels, and I do not have to take insulin.

I was seventy pounds overweight. My treatments for preventing diabetes and the use of a relatively unrestricted diet allowed me to bring my weight down to near-normal.

I used to look twenty years older than my actual age, yet I now look twenty years younger than my actual age.

I am 78 and believe I will live past 100.

Am I living on borrowed time?

No. I am taking advantage of new technologies to fix each health problem as it appears, and I am therefore dramatically improving my health and longevity.

The causes of aging and age-related diseases are finally being understood.

Dr. Rudman ran a series of tests on aging people and demonstrated that the effects of aging could be slowed and even reversed. He concluded: "The overall deterioration of the body that comes with growing old is not inevitable."

Tens of millions die from age-related conditions each and every year. That is because they think that it is natural to get old and die. They do not know about or do not take advantage of the programs that can already slow the processes and effects of degenerative aging.

America, and indeed the world, is aging. As the Baby Boomers continue to retire over the next several years they will significantly change society. Their diseases that come with aging will drastically affect the healthcare industry. But each of us can do something about it.

Aging Is Preventable.

You need to learn what you can do today to begin to slow your aging and to make sure that you live long enough to take advantage of all the future medical innovations now in the works.

You have choices of what you can do.

Understand and put into practice a basic, proven anti-aging program specifically tailored for you. The future of medicine is in personal tailoring.

Live Healthy - Look Marvelous - Live Longer

Aging is Preventable

Chapter 1
A Bit of History

"Study the past if you would define the future."
Confucius

To live young forever has been man's quest throughout history. From among the first writings preserved in the clay tablets of Babylon we read of King Gilgamesh who searched for the secret of eternal life.

The tablets tell us that he found it, but he lost it to the snake and then died.

Ponce de Leon searched for the fountain of youth, and he never found it.

My interest in finding a way to slow aging began many years ago. I made a film at Universal Studios about Ponce de Leon's Spring.

I describe the making of the film in my forthcoming book: The Spring of Eternity.

Picture from my Universal Studios Film: The Spring

Almost all life on earth blossoms with youth until it has reproduced and passed its genes on to the next generation. After that and a brief time to rear our young, Mother Nature has no further use for us, so we age and die.

But we are now beginning to understand aging. Medical science and the unraveling of the human genome have, and are, providing us with great insights into how our bodies work and how we are susceptible to diseases and the aging process.

Our new understandings now allow us to significantly increase our healthy longevity. And when we take advantages of these new findings we may live longer and thereby make ourselves available to take advantages of the even newer technologies being developed.

It is strongly believed by many researchers that our continuing progress will lead to the elimination of the disease of aging.

Some notable steps towards our understanding of the aging process have been made. Consider the following.

Discovery of the Double Helix of DNA

James Watson and Francis Crick discovered the model of DNA's double-helical structure in 1953. The knowledge we gained from understanding this detailed structure was critical to the development of age prevention programs.

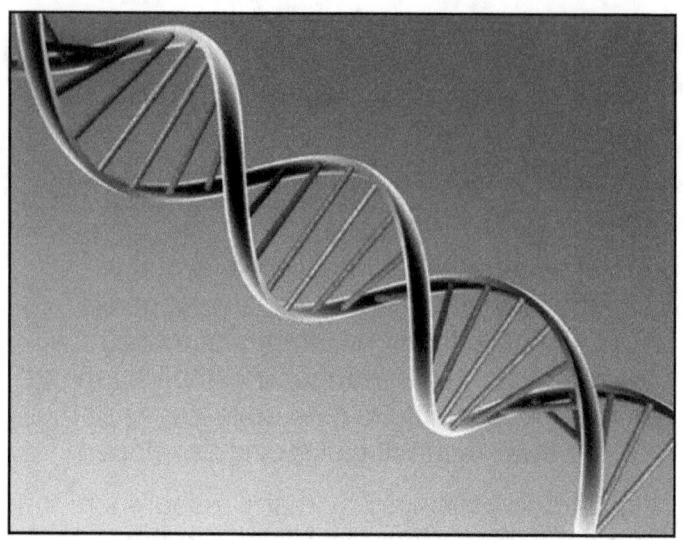

Discovery of the Telomere Death Clock

Dr. Hayflick discovered our built-in death clock in 1961 when he discovered the telomeres at the ends of the chromosomes.

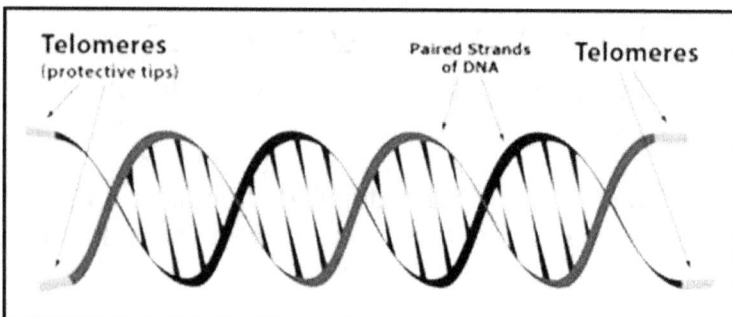

He described how they keep the chromosome organized but then erode each time our cells divide to replace old, inoperative cells. He learned that our telomeres have a limited number of times to allow cells to divide and replace themselves.

Dr. Hayflick determined that telomere erosion over time limits our lifespan to 120 years if disease or accidents do not get us earlier. The erosion occurs when the cells split to reproduce themselves. This limited number of reproductions is termed the Hayflick limit.

But far worst than limiting our life span, this death clock starts winding us down decades before it finally ends us. Long before the telomeres get too short for reproduction, the cells that they do reproduce with shortened telomeres are frequently weak and susceptible to disease. We begin the aging process.

I interviewed Dr. Hayflick several years ago to get his insight into this built-in death clock. He was convinced that we would never be able to live past 120 years because of our telomere erosion.

It should be noted that interestingly enough this 120 years is also the limit of life stated in the Bible: "And the LORD said, My spirit shall not always strive with man, for that he also is flesh: yet his days shall be an hundred and twenty years." Genesis 6.3

But as you will see below, this limitation of life can be removed.

Re-setting the Death Clock

In 1982 Blackburn and Szostak added to Dr. Hayflick's findings and presented their findings of how telomeres, the DNA caps on the end of chromosomes, protect our DNA chromosomes when cells divide.

Then in 1984 Greider and Blackburn identified telomerase, the enzyme that activates and makes telomere DNA.

Telomerase causes the telomeres to re-grow to replace the telomere length lost in the cell divisions.

Age prevention programs can now use telomerase to maintain telomere length so that healthy cell division can continue indefinitely.

Dr. Harley Makes Human Cells Immortal

Dr. Harley of the Geron Corporation used telomerase to make human cells immortal in the laboratory. I interviewed him after his successful experimental test. He was fearful that the use of telomerase might make the human cells cancerous because telomerase is the enzyme used by cancer cells to make themselves immortal.

Telomerase Does Not Cause Cancers

So cancer cells are basically immortal because they secrete their own telomerase. This led many to fear that the use of telomerase in anti-aging treatments would cause cancer.

Dr. Kaszubowska at the University of Gdansk Poland showed that centenarians have long telomeres and thereby proved that lengthening telomeres does not cause cancer.

Hormone Replacement

The first real evidence that we can take actions that can significantly affect our aging process began to be realizable in 1989 when Dr. Rudman ran hormone replacement experiments on twelve men, ages 61 to 81, and he compared them to an age-matched control group. He turned their flabby, frail, fat-bulging bodies into their sleeker, stronger, younger selves.

Rudman reported: *"The effects were equivalent in magnitude to the changes incurred during 10 to 20 years of aging."*

In effect he had reversed their biological ages by 10 to 20 years.

Dr. Rudman concluded: *"The overall deterioration of the body that comes with growing old is not inevitable."*

I experimented with Dr. Rudman's treatments and had great results. But I soon stopped because of fear of possible side effects.

I realized that the use of hormone precursor supplements as opposed to the use of hormone replacement per se was a much safer way to go. I will describe this technique later.

Dr. Chein Provided 10 to 20 Years of Age Reversal

Following Dr. Rudman's tests Dr. Chein used Hormone Replacement Therapy (HRT) with several hundred patients and reversed their biological ages by 10 to 20 years.

Human Genome Decoded

The complete Human Genome was decoded in 2003, allowing us to better understand our genetic structure.

Dr. Xu Shows That Multivitamins Activate the Telomerase Genes

Dr. Xu and his group at the National Institute of Health showed that the use of multivitamins is associated with longer telomere length.

Tests Prove That Telomerase Treatments can Prolong Life by 10 to 20 Years

Several tests by several different researchers, as described herein, prove that telomerase treatments can extend telomere length equivalent to an extra 10 to 20 years of life.

The Geron Corporation Develops Astragalus Membranaceus

The Geron Corporation develops Astragalus Membranaceus and conduct tests, with others, to prove that it can activate the telomerase gene and significantly extend life.

Three Scientists Win the 2009 Nobel Prize in Medicine for Telomerase

Three scientists, Elizabeth H. Blackburn, PhD, of University of California, San Francisco and Carol W. Greider, PhD, of Johns Hopkins University School of Medicine and Jack W. Szostak, PhD, of Massachusetts General Hospital, Harvard Medical School and Howard Hughes Medical Institute jointly win the 2009 Nobel Prize in Medicine for discovering how telomerase works to lengthen the telomere portion of our DNA.

They showed how telomerase achieves youthful cell replications and perpetual non-dying cells in the laboratory.

***

We are entering a new era of anti-aging medicine that has been proven to slow aging.

Chapter 2

Understanding Our DNA Structure

"I think that the formation of [DNA's] structure by Watson and Crick may turn out to be the greatest developments in the field of molecular genetics in recent years."

Linus Pauling

Now with better understanding of the prevention of telomere shortening via telomerase, we can use telomerase activation ingredients, including hormone precursors and other nutracuetials that have been proven to do the following:

1. Slow telomere erosion

2. Rebuild telomeres

3. Prevent biological aging

4. Reverse biological aging

To understand how this works you need to understand the DNA structure of our chromosomes and telomeres.

DNA is a double stranded helix made up of base pairs. It is frequently depicted as follows:

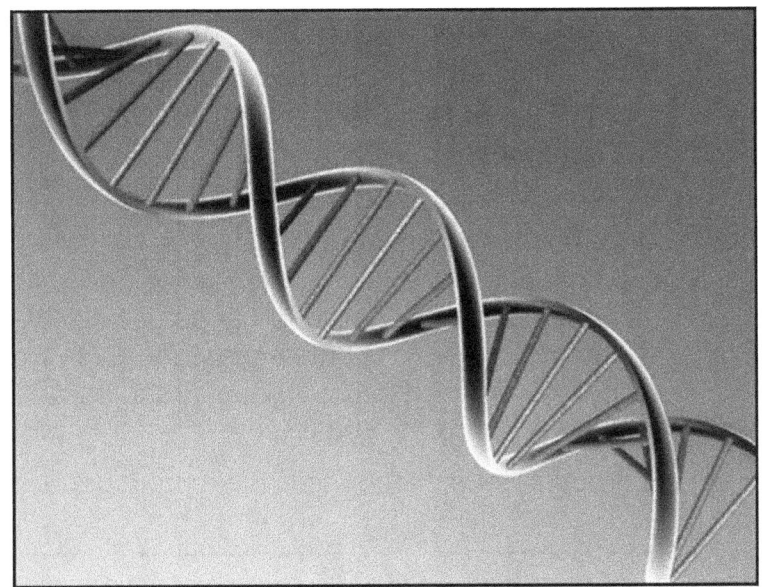

We need to take a closer look to better understand.

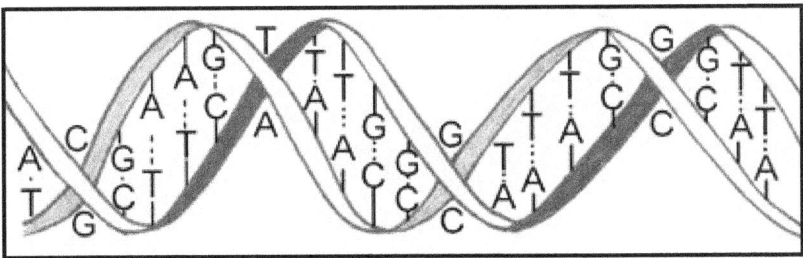

The base pairs, i.e. the "steps in the DNA ladder" are made of 4 substances: adenine on one strand always pairs with thymine on the other strand. These are called A-T pairs, regardless of which strand has the "A" and which the "T."

Similarly, cytosine on one strand always pairs with guanine on the other strand, creating G-C pairs.

Scientists often represent DNA strands with a string of letters like this:

ATATTTGAAAGCTGTGTCTGTAAACTGATG GCTAACAAAACTAG.

This string of letters represents only one strand, or one-half of the DNA molecule. There is no need to write down the other strand because as we just described, a "G" in one strand means there is automatically a "C" in the other strand, just as a "C" in one strand implies that the other contains a "G."

A group of these sequences make up a gene as illustrated.

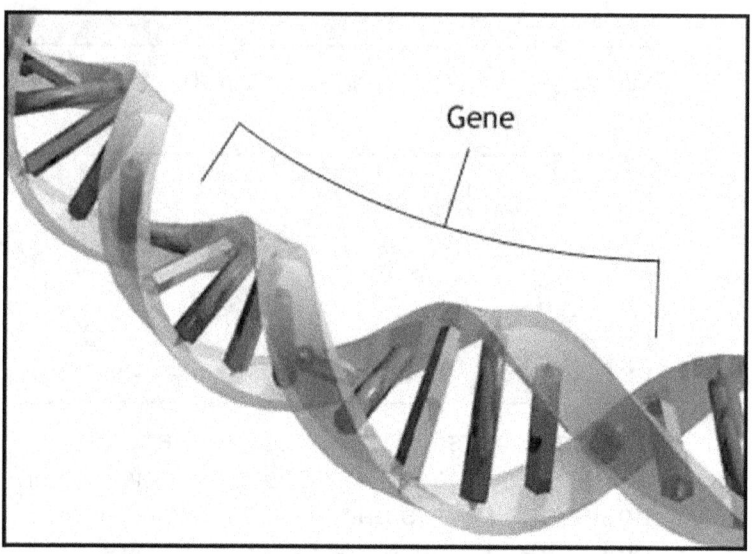

Gene

The average gene is about 27,000 base pairs long. The longest yet discovered is a muscle-production gene that is 3.2 billion base pairs long.

At the end of each chromosome are telomeres, which are non-coding repeating genes with the base pair sequence of TTAGGG. The telomere can reach a length of 15,000 base pairs.

Telomeres function by preventing chromosomes from losing base pair sequences at their ends. They also stop chromosomes from fusing to each other. However, each time a cell divides to replace itself, some of the telomere, usually about 25-200 base pairs per division, is lost.

When the telomere becomes too short, the chromosome reaches a critical length and can no longer replicate. This means that its cell becomes too old and dies without being able to replace itself.

Preventing Aging

We can stop aging by preventing telomere erosion, or alternatively by re-growing the telomere length.

The key to preventing telomere erosion is in reactivating our genes that produce telomerase.

Telomerase

Our bodies naturally produce an enzyme called telomerase that prevents telomere erosion while we are babies in the womb. This is necessary to accommodate the large number of cell divisions required for our rapid growth while in the womb.

Our bodies produce very little telomerase after birth and then only to accommodate our continuing rapid growth until age four or five.

Thereafter we produce essentially no meaningful levels of telomerase.

But the mechanism for the production of telomerase remains coded in our DNA that is in almost all of our cells. However, the signal to activate the mechanism, i.e. turn on the coding for telomerase, is no longer active.

If we could turn this signal back on we could stop our internal biological aging clock. We could theoretically live forever until we encounter a non-aging form of death.

We have not yet found a way to fully turn our "death clock" off, but we have found ways to partially activate the clock in a manner to slow down the aging process, and we have developed evidence that we will soon be able to turn if off completely.

Making Human Cells Immortal

The Geron Corporation has used telomerase to make human cells immortal in the lab. We therefore know that it is possible. It's just a matter of time until telomerase treatments can become routine.

Chapter 3

Understanding the Causes of Aging

"You can't help getting older, but you don't have to get old." George Burns

Okay, so now you have a basic understanding of our DNA structure. Next you need to understand some of the fundamentals about aging and anti-aging.

Medical science and the unraveling of the human genome have, and are, providing us with great insights into how our bodies work and how we are susceptible to diseases and the aging process.

Our new understandings allow us to significantly increase our healthy longevity. And when we take advantages of these new findings we have the opportunity to take advantage of even more that are being developed for the future.

So the idea is to take advantage of each new anti-aging development and to be alive so we can continue this process until we become immortal.

Really? Stay with me and see if you agree.

To understand the causes of aging we need to recognize just what our primary purpose here on earth really is: we were designed by God or Mother Nature, depending on your religious views, to perpetuate the species of Man here on Earth.

After we have matured and passed our genes on to our children we are designed to then only live long enough to rear our young. After that Mother Nature has no reason to keep us around, so we age and die.

We age because the products of our metabolism, i.e., the ashes from the oxidation processes that produce energy in our cells, accumulate faster than our aging endocrine systems can remove them. This is because most of the cleansing hormones that surged through our youthful bodies begin to decrease as we begin to age. Some of these more critical hormones have decreased by about 10 to 30 percent as we enter our thirties.

The decreases become ever-more dramatic as we enter successive decades of life. Most of our hormones have decreased by over 50%, and some have been reduced to near zero as we enter our seventies.

So we age.

Our muscles and bones weaken; our reaction times slow; we lose our agility. All of this combines to make us more susceptible to accidents. Our immune system weakens and makes us more susceptible to disease.

And we die.

And even worst, superimposed on these causes of aging and death is the built-in inevitability of death: our built-in telomere erosion death clock previously described.

Let's look a little closer at the causes of aging.

There are a dozen or so mechanisms of aging that have been theorized over time. I believe that there are six primary causes that combine to make us age:

1. Free radicals: Lipofuscins and other ashes of our metabolism and environmental toxins build up in our cells and cause the cells to die without being able to reproduce as they would normally do when you are younger.

2. Hormone Decline: Our endocrine system ceases to secrete sufficient quantities of certain enzymes and hormones to keep up with the cells' battles with the build up of contaminants.

3. Telomere Erosion: Our cells lose their abilities to divide and replace themselves because they use up their allotted number of divisions.

4. Stress: Causes secretion of excessive cortisol, which does significant damages and make us age more rapidly.

5. Diet Deficiencies and Excesses: Limits the materials necessary for the cells to cleanse and repair themselves. Excesses in our diets adversely affect certain chemical reactions.

6. Lack of Exercise: Causes atrophy of critical muscles that result in chemical imbalances in our endocrine system and loss of strength and agility, which makes us prone to accidents.

Some people have also inherited flawed genes that may affect aging. We have developed treatments to replace defective genes with some success.

The first treatment occurred in 1999, and many more treatments have occurred since. All of these have been experimental and conducted by researchers. It will be a while longer before the procedures will be available to the general public.

Let's review more details about the six primary causes.

1. Free Radicals, Lipofuscins, and Toxins

Mitochondria, located in almost all of your cells, convert the food you eat into energy.

The mitochondrion is a sausage-shaped, double-membrane organelle appropriately nicknamed the cell's powerhouse because of its efficiency in converting food into a form of energy called ATP.

This conversion to energy leaves a residue of ashes from the oxidation process that produces energy in our cells.

In addition to the build up of these ashes, there are additional adverse side effects. In the process, i.e. burning the food with oxygen, unwanted free oxygen radicals are generated. These radicals are a form of oxygen that wants to keep on burning with something.

These free radical molecules cause dangerous inflammation in the cell. They attack the insides of the cell, its walls, and even its DNA. This eventually will cause the cell to become inoperative and die.

This oxidation is analogous to rusting. It results in a rusting of your arteries, which is partly responsible for the aging of your cardiovascular system.

Lipofuscins are the brown age spots we see on our aging skin. Similar spots and contaminates accumulate in our heart muscles, brains, and elsewhere.

Further, various types of environmental toxins find their way into our cells and frequently behave as free radicals and/or accumulate to the point of clogging the cell and impeding its operation.

Some of the toxins that we encounter are potentially very harmful and can cause cancer, asthma, various allergies, and can significantly reduce quality of life. Their affects tend to speed up the aging process.

Our bodies naturally combat these processes by providing anti-oxidants from the food we eat and supplements that we may take. Such anti-oxidants include the well-known vitamins C and E that we get by eating certain fruits and vegetables and by supplementation.

And there are many more free radical fighters in the form of many dozens of other anti-oxidants and nutrients. The best fighters are the enzymes and hormones described below.

But we lose our best fighters as we age, and the free radicals eventually win their battles.

We age and die.

But we can do something about free radicals as described later.

2. Hormone and Enzyme Decline

Our hormones regulate and control most of the functions of our bodies. Testosterone and estrogen, the major sex hormones in men and women respectively, give us the urge and ability to reproduce and continue the survival of our species.

But once we're past our reproductive prime, our hormone levels drop. This results in a lack of sex drive, insomnia, impotence, weight gain, and countless other potential health problems that significantly decrease our quality of life.

So we see that our hormone system was designed primarily for reproduction for the survival of the species. Our bodies produce high quantities of certain hormones and enzymes during our youth. These give us our youthful vitality, strength, and endurance. They help in the battles against free radicals, and they help provide nutrients for cell repair. They keep our cells cleansed of the ashes of metabolism and environmental toxins.

As long as our bodies produce sufficient quantities of these enzymes and hormones, we stay young.

As we age past our prime reproductive years we are no longer capable of producing sufficient quantities of the enzymes and hormones required to keep our cells young and fit. With too little of these substances, our cells begin to lose their battles against the free radicals and other destructive elements.

The cells begin to age and die. The organs of which they are a part become ineffective. We become frail, and we die.

But we can do something about hormonal decline as is described in a later chapter.

3. Telomere Erosion

Telomere erosion is the primary factor that, even if all other factors are cured, will eventually lead to death.

Baring poor nutrition and a poor environment, the telomeres of most of our cells may allow replacement for up to the age approaching 120 years.

We can now use the information that we have learned to prevent, or at least slow telomere erosion as I describe in a later Chapter.

4. Stress

A study in 2004 first identified the direct link between stress and aging. Intense, long-term emotional strain and stress can make you sick and grow old much faster than normal.

Stress is a normal part of life. Almost everything that happens to us puts stress on our bodies. You can experience stress from your environment, actions or inactions, the actions or inaction of others, body aches, and even just your thoughts.

The human body is designed to experience stress and to react to it. Stress has a positive side in that it keeps us alert and ready to avoid danger. Stress becomes negative when you face continuous challenges without relief or relaxation between said challenges. As a result, stress-related tension builds.

Our adrenalin system was designed to handle acute stress, which is experienced in response to an immediately perceived threat, such as a lion about to eat us. During an acute stress response, the autonomic nervous system is activated, and the body experiences increased levels of cortisol, adrenalin, and other hormones that produce an increased heart rate, quickened breathing rate, and higher blood pressure. Blood is shunted to the big muscles to prepare the body to fight or run away.

This is commonly known as the fight-or-flight response.

But our lives have changed. Now we are more likely to be subjected to chronic stress, which our bodies are not designed to handle.

Many of us experience chronic stresses caused by our modern lifestyle. It can be caused by everything from high-pressured jobs to loneliness to traffic. Such chronic stress can keep the body in a state of perceived threat. When this happens, our fight-or-flight response, which was designed to help us fight a few life-threatening situations spaced out over a long period, can wear down our bodies and cause us to become ill, physically or emotionally.

Chronic stress, sometimes termed distress, causes negative kinds of stress reactions. It occurs when stress continues without any relief. Distress can lead to physical symptoms including headaches, upset stomach, elevated blood pressure, chest pain, and insomnia.

Research shows that stress can also cause or worsen some diseases.

Stress causes the release of the so-called stress hormones, of which cortisol is the primary. Chronically elevated levels of cortisol speeds up the shortening of the telomeres and causes the cells to become ineffective in carrying out their purposes. As previously described, we know that shortened telomeres speeds the body's deterioration and causes aging.

Cells with shortened telomeres cannot divide to form new cells, so the cells die without replacing themselves. The tissue to which the cells are a part of then ages much more quickly and soon dies.

And then we die.

So stress prematurely shortens our telomeres and speeds up aging.

This helps explain the association between psychological stress and increased risk of physical disease. Unrelenting emotional pressure and stress definitely accelerates the aging process.

But we can do something to relieve chronic stress as described in a later chapter.

5. Dietary Deficiencies and Excesses

Most of us in today's more advanced societies do not experience dietary deficiencies unless or until we get older. But how fast and how well we age will be affected when and if we do experience such deficiencies.

Our diets consist of five nutritional groups:

1. Proteins

2. Carbohydrates

3. Fats

4. Vitamins

5. Minerals

There are about 50 nutritional items within these groups that are necessary for good health. Age, gender, and overall health dictate how much of each of these nutrients we need.

We need to insure that we get all of the nutrients that we need from each of the five groups to prevent any deficiencies. Relatively simple blood tests can determine any deficiencies and can monitor for any developing deficiencies.

Diet excesses can also adversely affect health and the aging process. Excesses and obesity can cause basic changes in our body's chemistry.

When deficiencies and excesses exist they can be treated by diet changes and with supplements.

6. Lack of Exercise

We all well know that lack of exercise causes muscle atrophy, which results in loss of strength and agility and makes us prone to accidents. It is less known that this atrophy can result in chemical imbalances that degrade our immune systems and make us more susceptible to diseases.

And perhaps most important, insufficient exercise can cause our telomeres to shorten at a faster rate.

Chapter 4
Understanding Hormones

"Every patient carries his or her own doctor inside."

Albert Schweitzer

Okay, so we understand the causes of aging. Now let's understand how our hormones work.

Our hormones regulate and control most of the functions of our bodies. I have summarized how our hormones and enzymes work in the above discussion about the causes of aging.

As long as our bodies produce sufficient quantities of these enzymes and hormones, we stay young. But as we age past our prime reproductive years we are no longer capable of producing sufficient quantities of the enzymes and hormones required to keep our cells "young and fit."

Let's review a little more detail for each of the key hormones:

Human Growth Hormone (HGH)

Testosterone

Estrogen

Progesterone

DHEA

Melatonin

Pregnenolone

Thymus Hormones

Thyroid Hormone

Insulin

Stress Hormones

Chapter 4.1 Human Growth Hormone (HGH)

Human Growth Hormone (HGH) is the master hormone of the body and is therefore the principle hormone in anti-aging and other hormone replacement therapies (HRT) and hormone precursor therapies (HPT).

HGH is a protein hormone, not a steroid. The somatotropic cells of the anterior lobe of the pituitary gland secrete it. Its technical name is somatotropin. It is secreted in pulses throughout the 24-hour day, with the major secretions occurring during the beginning phases of sleep.

HGH directs and supports the other hormones and thereby affects all glands and organs in the body. HGH is the body's most essential maintenance and repair hormone, and like testosterone, it has major anabolic, i.e. muscle building, effects.

Adequate HGH levels are required for:

Cell replacement

Tissue Repair

Healing

Bone Strength

Brain function

Organ integrity

Enzyme protection

Integrity of hair nails and skin

Re-activation of telomerase genes

Our chief problem with HGH and several of the key hormones is that the body's natural secretion of hormones rapidly declines with age. By sixty, we have less than 40% of the values we had at twenty. The following chart shows the decreases for three of the key hormones.

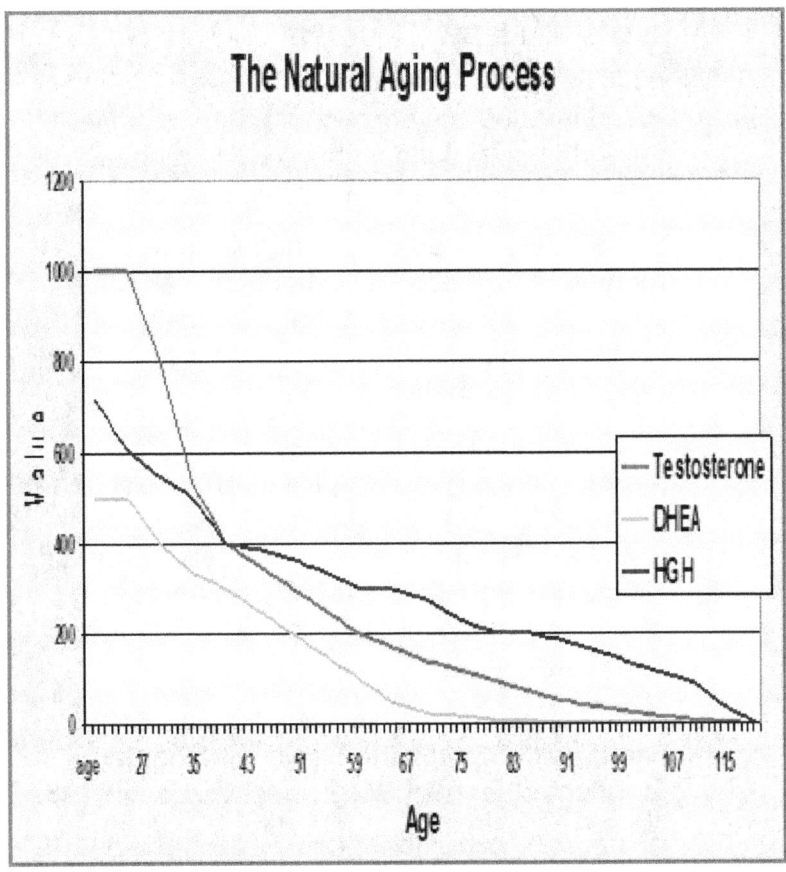

It should be noted that HGH is difficult to measure because of its variability during each 24-hour period. It is therefore measured indirectly by measuring insulin-like growth factor-I (IGF-I). IGF-I is typically between 300 and 450 ng/nl (nanograms per milliliter of blood) for healthy young adults.

It declines with HGH as we age, at the rate of about 10 to 15 percent per decade. In older people it therefore ranges from 30 to 200. Many in the anti-aging community consider values below 350 a deficiency.

1) HGH History and Tests

HGH was discovered in the 1920s and first used in 1958 on a growth-stunted boy. He grew taller, and since then HGH has become the common treatment for this disorder.

Initially, HGH was only available from cadavers. In 1985 Genentech spliced human DNA into bacteria, and the genetically engineered bacteria began producing HGH at an affordable price.

Eli Lilly engineered a more exact replica of HGH with the genetic splicing of human genes in bacteria. This produced an HGH of the precise 191 amino acids produced by normal humans – versus the 190 amino acids of the earlier synthetic. Eli Lilly is now the leader in HGH supply.

The limitations imposed by cadaver sources were quickly eliminated, and Dr. Rudman conducted tests of HGH effectiveness in 1989.

During a six-month test on 12 men aged 61-81 (against a control group of 9 men); the men lost 14.4% of their body fat and gained 8.8% lean body mass. Their skin thickened, their bone density increased, and their livers and spleens increased to youthful sizes.

Dr. Rudman showed that HGH could change flabby, frail old men aged 61- 81 back to their previous biological ages of 41-61. In effect, he reversed their ages by 20 years over a six-month period.

He concluded: "The overall deterioration of the body that comes with growing old is not inevitable."

In his follow up six-month study with the same men, their muscle masses increased an additional 6% (over the original 8.8%), and they lost an additional 15% fat (after the original 14.4% loss).

Others have repeated Dr. Rudman's tests and found similar results. There was a cry for the FDA to approve it as an anti-aging therapy, but the FDA only approved it for stunted-growth children.

Nevertheless, it hit the black market and began to be widely used by bodybuilders and others.

Then in 1991, Texas businessman Howard Turney opened El Dorado Rejuvenation Clinic in Mexico, beyond control of the FDA.

Then in 1994, Dr. Edmund Chein found a loophole in the FDA restriction. He went to court and argued that since the FDA had approved HGH for stunted-growth disorder that then a certified physician should be able to prescribe it for any purpose he sees fit. He won his argument and opened Palm Springs Life Extension Institute in California.

He has since treated thousands of people between the ages of 31 and 92 to slow, stop, or reverse their aging. He has succeeded with most. And he reports no significant adverse side effects during any of his operations.

Chein's results in increased muscle mass were 10.0% and 8.0% increase for two six-month periods, similar to Dr. Rudman's results.

HGH makes fat more available as a fuel. Fat cells have hormone receptors that trigger a host of enzymatic reactions when HGH is present.

HGH has also been shown to enhance the effectiveness of the immune system. One major way it does this is to increase the thymus gland's output of T-cells (that destroy invading germs). This is especially important for people over 40. The thymus normally shrinks to the size of a raisin by age 40 (See: Thymus Factors in a later section).

Tests also indicate that HGH can reverse heart disease by thickening the walls of the weakened ventricles.

Tests have shown that HGH also improves LDL/HDL cholesterol ratios. It can prevent osteoporosis and even reverse it. It can improve vision, increase clarity of thought, improve or restore sexual functions, and re-grow hair.

Dr. Sam Boxas of Switzerland uses HGH to treat muscular sclerosis, lupus, Alzheimer's, Lou Gehrig's disease, and even AIDS. And, as unbelievable as it sounds, he says: "We are healing just about everything."

He is effectively reversing aging.

Several doctors have reported that HGH has resulted in their patients showing a marked progressiveness towards homeostasis, i.e. body balance. Everyone experienced higher metabolism and more youthful body chemistry. Their DHEA was generally up by 33%, and the male's testosterone levels were up an average of 18.5%. Cholesterol was down an average of 14.8%, and triglycerides were down 31%.

The patients generally reported the following qualitative improvements:

Weight reduction

Muscle increase

Energy up

Libido up

Skin rejuvenation

Hair color return

Greater hair density

Improved mental stability

There were no significant adverse side effects reported. These early tests with HGH strongly indicated that HGH could restore youth safely.

2) Benefits of HGH HRT and HPT

The early tests plus the many follow up tests have shown that HGH HRT and HPT can provide the following benefits:

Improved immune function

Accelerates wound healing

Strengthen bones

Reverse osteoporosis

Reverse muscle wasting

Increase muscle mass

Decrease fat

Eliminate cellulite

Reduce appetite

Increase exercise performance

Lower blood pressure

Lower bad cholesterol

Increase good HDL

Lower triglycerides

Increase cardiac output

Restore the size of heart, liver, pancreas, kidneys, spleen, and other organs that had shrunk with age

Enhance collagen synthesis and repair

Provide tighter, more hydrated, smoother, and thicker skin

Improve brain function

Improve cognitive abilities

Improve memory and concentration

Grow neuron dendrites to repair brain injury or treat disease

Improve vision

Provide higher energy levels

Achieve less fatigue and less depression

Reduce stress levels

Elevate mood

Improve quality of deep sleep

Enhance sexuality, drive, and performance

Reduce accumulation of lipofuscins

Prevent chronic, degenerative diseases

Reverse the effects of aging.

Dr. Ronald Klatz, President of the American Academy of Anti-Aging, and author of the book Grow Young with HGH, summarizes the benefits of HGH replacement therapy in the following statement:

"HGH is the ultimate anti-aging therapy. It affects every cell in the body, rejuvenating the skin and bones, regenerating the heart, liver, lung, and kidneys, bringing organ and tissue function back to youthful levels. It is the most effective anti-obesity agent ever discovered, revving up the metabolism to youthful levels, re-sculpturing the body by selectively reducing the fat in the waist, abdomen, hips, thighs, and at the same time increasing muscle mass. It may be the most powerful aphrodisiac ever discovered, reviving flagging sexuality and potency in men and women. It is cosmetic surgery in a bottle, smoothing out facial wrinkles; restoring the elasticity, thickness and contours of youthful skin; reversing the loss of

extra cellular water that makes old people look like dried-up old prunes. It has healing powers that close ulcerated wounds and re-grow burned skin. It reverses the insomnia of later life, restoring "slow wave" or the deepest level of sleep. And, it is a mood elevator, lifting the spirit along with the body, bringing back a zest for life that many people thought was long gone."

Dr. Edmund Chein, one of the first providers of HGH replacement therapy, is more succinct: *"It's a slam dunk! This (HGH) is 100% effective!"*

3) HGH and the Immune System

If there is one aspect of our metabolism that simply must function effectively to ensure one's survival, it is the immune system. It has to defend us against the nasty world of microbes and viruses as well as parasites that are continuously invading our bodies. We survive their assault when our immune system works optimally.

But as we age, so does our immune system. One of the major glands of our immune system is our thymus. In childhood, this gland creates T-lymphocytes, the specialized cells that eliminate bacteria, viruses, and foreign matter from our bodies.

In late childhood, the thymus is the size of a plum, but at puberty it begins to shrink. By the time we reach old age it's no larger than a small raisin.

This atrophication of the thymus parallels the decline of our immune system.

HGH can regenerate the thymus and restore our immune system to near the optimum function that it had when we were twelve years old. The statisticians have shown that this is the age we are least likely to die from disease.

Tests on dogs in 1980 showed that when growth hormone replacement was instituted, "The thymuses of growth-hormone-treated dogs regenerated, resembling thymic tissue of young dogs."

In 1991, David Khansari and Thomas Gustad of North Dakota State University completed a long-term study on mice. They divided 52 mice that had reached the age of senescence (old age) into two equal groups.

One group was given growth hormone for 13 weeks. Most of these members were still living after all the members of the control group had died. It was also noted that the growth-hormone-treated mice had T-cell counts comparable to those of young mice. With their newly empowered immune systems, they lived beyond the normal limit for mice.

Scientists at University of New Mexico School of Medicine took twelve older women in relatively good health but with low HGH levels, and they gave six of them HGH for fourteen days. The six treated women experienced a 20% increase in their T- cell activity compared to the untreated women.

HGH can obviously regenerate the thymus gland and vastly improve the immune system.

4) HGH and the Brain

HGH is one of the few substances that cross the blood-brain barrier.

Tests have shown that there are receptor sights for HGH in numerous parts of the brain, including the hypothalamus, the pituitary, and the hippocampus. The receptors in the hippocampus are of particular interest because this is a part of the brain that significantly controls cognitive functions and memory.

This recognition has made HGH a source of hope in treating Alzheimer's disease and memory-related diseases of our aging population.

One third to one half of all 85-year-olds are at least in the early stages of Alzheimer's disease. Dr. Chaovanee Aroonsakul of the Alzheimer's and Parkinson's disease Diagnostic and Treatment Center in Naperville, Illinois, has reported noticeable improvements after treatment with HGH in both these conditions as well as in patients suffering other forms of senile dementia.

In a study of over three hundred subjects, Dr. Aroonsakul reported consistently lower levels of HGH in patients with Parkinson's and multiple sclerosis, as well as stroke patients, and she found profound deficiency of HGH in Alzheimer's patients.

Dr. Aroonsakul has reported some improvement in Alzheimer's patients after several years of continuous HGH therapy. She believes that HGH improves cerebral blood flow, revitalizes neuronal dendrites and axons, and enhances repair of proteins in the brain, causing an increase in the formation of RNA and DNA.

5) HGH and the Bones

Tens of millions of Americans suffer serious, crippling damage to their bones; this leads elderly people to nursing homes more than any other cause.

We lose bone mass and density as we age because of hormonal declines. It begins in our thirties when androgen levels start to decline. Bone is a hormonally sensitive tissue.

The major disease of the bones is osteoporosis, which literally means "porous bones." It is perhaps the most expensive and debilitating disease in America.

Osteoporosis is a chronic degenerative bone disease that over time causes an excessive loss of bone. Osteoporosis is like a termite infestation. You don't know you have it until something breaks.

Once in their forties, most people lose bone at the rate of 0.5% per year. For women, this increases by a factor of ten after menopause. Many women lose a third of their bone mass before the age of sixty. Half of all women have an osteoporosis fracture by the age of seventy.

Twenty percent of osteoporosis patients are men, and their problems usually come later than for women.

Twenty-four million Americans have osteoporosis and collectively spend $10 billion per year treating it or dealing with its consequences.

In a healthy and young body, bones are continuously being torn down and rebuilt. Each year about 25% of a typical bone is dismantled, i.e. reabsorbed, and then replaced.

Osteoclasts are the cells that serve as the demolition crew. Osteoblasts are the reconstruction crew. Osteoblasts build new bone continuously by depositing calcium phosphate on the protein framework of existing bone.

The bones are built up to the level of their maximum density and health by the time we are in our twenties. They then begin a slight decline in our mid-thirties.

For those of us who want to live a long, healthy life, we need a bone survival plan.

Both HGH and testosterone (as described later) stimulate Osteoblasts to halt and reverse bone loss. HGH and the principal androgens, including testosterone, scavenge available calcium from the blood and put it back into the bone.

Therefore, our bone survival plan requires proper levels of dietary (or supplemental) calcium and proper levels of hormones that know how to put that calcium where it will do the most good.

This plan will vary from individual to individual depending on their individual health profile and dietary habits. As an example, those ingesting high quantities of sugar will need more calcium and hormones because sugar depletes our bodies of calcium. Salt and caffeine also increase our excretion of calcium within a few hours of consumption.

Phosphorus also adversely affects our bone health. Soda beverages that are high in caffeine, sugar, and phosphorus are absolutely the worst drinks possible for bone health.

Cola drinkers will need special doses of HGH.

6) Benefits of HGH HRT and HPT

Perhaps the best quantifiable summary of the benefits of HGH HRT is that by Dr. Chein and Dr. Terry from their six-month test of 202 subjects. These patients each gave personal assessments of the results of their treatments. Their personal assessments were combined with other results from tests by others - as previously described - which indicate many more benefits. Unfortunately, some of the tests were not of a quantifiable nature.

The resulting summary of the benefits of HGH HRT is presented in Chapter 7 below.

7) Adverse Side Effects of HGH HRT

Fluid retention was the most common side effect reported. All reported, however, that it was a very transient effect that ceased after a day or two. Even this transient effect was shown to be avoidable by starting patients at lower dosages and then ramping them up to the desired dose over time.

Some patients reported acne. Ramping also eliminated this side effect.

Arthralgia (joint pain) was reported in a few cases (0.7%). Again, down ramping eliminated the problem.

Carpal tunnel syndrome was also reported in a few cases (0.5%) and was also eliminated by down ramping.

Other researchers have also reported these side effects, plus gynecomastia and painful cartilage growth. But in all cases reported, the doses were much higher than the doses used and recommended by doctors working in the area.

There has also been some concern expressed by some critics that HGH replacement therapy could increase the probability of some cancers, especially the spreading of cancers already existing when therapy is initiated. The primary cancers of concern were breast and prostate cancers.

But, on the contrary, tests by Dr. Terry showed that some existing cancers went into remission when HGH therapy was used!

Dr. Terry said, *"It is mind boggling."*

He does not know why the remission occurred. Dr. Chein speculates that the growth hormone stimulated the immune system, increasing the natural killer cells, which effectively destroyed the cancer cells.

Another concern is that the pituitary gland may reduce its secretion of HGH when HGH is given externally, i.e. by replacement therapy. I also have this concern.

Dr. George Merriam at the University of Washington in Seattle conducted a study on growth hormone for the National Institute of Aging (NIA), and concluded the following: ***"There is no evidence suggesting that this (growth Hormone) replacement therapy causes any unfavorable long term side effects; a complete absence of side effects."***

Nevertheless, I believe that HRT is too risky and that there is a safer way to go. I suggest the use of Hormone Precursor Therapy (HPT) as opposed to HRT. HPT uses FDA approved nutracuetials as precursors to HGH, as described later. These precursors stimulate the body to increase its own production of HGH.

8) HGH Summary

Proper levels of HGH are necessary for optimum health. The benefits are enormous. However there can be significant adverse affects for HRT. Therefore it is safer to use HPT because, though it is less effective, there are essentially no adverse side effects. Tests have shown that the recommended HGH precursors, taken properly, will return HGH levels towards more youthful levels and will, at least partially, re-activate the telomerase genes and slow aging.

Tests and test results are described in Chapter 7 below.

Chapter 4.2 Testosterone

Testosterone is the primary male sex hormone and is a secondary but very vital female sex hormone. Women produce it to the levels of about one tenth to one twelfth that of men.

Testosterone HRT and/or HPT are vital for anti-aging programs.

Testosterone is produced by the testicles in men and by the ovaries in women. It builds up in boys and causes the changes of puberty; it makes a male a male.

Estrogen is the principal female hormone that makes a female a female, but it is testosterone that triggers some of the secondary sex changes in females at puberty, and stimulates her sex drive.

Testosterone sets the sex drive in both men and women.

There are receptors for testosterone in every part of our bodies, from brain to toes. The sexual areas of our bodies are packed with testosterone receptors.

When a girl reaches puberty, it is testosterone that stimulates the growth of pubic hair and underarm hair. At the same time, there are testosterone receptors in the nipples of her developing breasts and a heavy concentration in the area of her vagina and clitoris. There is little or no arousal unless testosterone flows to those regions.

Testosterone is also vitally involved in the making of protein, which in turn, forms muscle.

And testosterone is a key player in the manufacturing of bone.

Testosterone improves oxygen uptake throughout the body, thus vitalizing all tissues. Testosterone helps:

Control Blood Sugar

Regulate Cholesterol

Maintain a Powerful Immune System

Mental Concentration

Improve Mood

Protect Against Alzheimer's disease

Partially re-activate the telomerase genes

Biologically active testosterone drops rapidly with age as is shown in the previous chart. For many men, the drop after age 40 is even more drastic than the norm shown in the chart. This is generally the case for over 20% of men over the age of fifty.

The female production of free testosterone drops in the same fashion as men until their ovaries shut down at menopause. Thereafter their body usually converts a small amount of testosterone from DHEA. This amount is usually insufficient for normal, youthful body functions.

When testosterone gets below a certain level, there is a profound effect on physical health and well-being.

Specific symptoms are:

Loss of libido in both sexes

Inability to maintain an erection in men

Fatigue, irritability, depressed mood

Aches and pains in joints

Dry skin

Osteoporosis

Muscle loss

Hair loss

The natural decrease in our production of testosterone can occur sooner with the presence of any of the following factors:

Illness

Medication

Obesity

Lack of exercise

Poor psychological state

Smoking

Excessive Alcohol

Diabetes

Nutritional deficiency

Human Growth Hormone (HGH) deficiency

1) The Male Andropause

The lower levels of free testosterone for men, whether occurring with the decrease over time as depicted in the chart, or whether resulting from the 20% or so abnormalities, eventually cause all males to experience a male menopause. This is sometimes referred to as an "Andropause" or a "change of life" or "the male climacteric."

It is not as sudden as the female menopause. It may typically occur over a period of fifteen years or so. And it starts at different times for different men, some as early as the 40s, some as late as the 80s.

Arguments as to the occurrence of the male Andropause still continue, even though Dr. Carl Heller and Dr. Gordon Myers published the first proof in the Journal of the American Medical Association over fifty years ago.

They compared 38 men with "mid-life symptoms" with 25 healthy men. 23 of the 38 men had low testosterone levels. A 25 mg injection of testosterone was given to all the men five times per week for a period of two to four weeks. By the second week there were definite improvements in all the 23 men who had initially tested low in testosterone.

When testosterone was later withheld, their "mid-life symptoms" returned. It was concluded that the male Andropause did exist and that it could be treated with testosterone replacement. This replacement is typically referred to as Hormone Replacement Therapy (HRT).

2) Testosterone HRT and HPT for Men

Testosterone levels for optimal sex for men vary over very large ranges. The optimum level is directly related to the normal for the individual. Men with very high testosterone levels in their youth may experience sexual problems with drops to levels still as high as 500 micrograms per deciliter of blood, while men with low levels of testosterone in their youth will have excellent sexual function at a level of 500.

Testosterone HRT may be administered by intra-muscular injections, via patches, or by the applications of creams, with the best method being dependent on the individual.

Testosterone HPT is not as fast-acting or as effective as HRT. But it is safer and does not conflict with the government's effective band on HRT for anti-aging.

3) Testosterone HRT and HPT for Women

Testosterone is not just for men. Testosterone, the quintessential male hormone, is also a female hormone.

Healthy women naturally have small amounts of testosterone in their bodies. In fact, the female reproductive organs, the ovaries, produce it.

As with estrogen and progesterone, a woman's testosterone levels drop as she ages. A woman could be diligently taking her estrogen and progesterone each day, and she may still not feel like herself. That is because she is ignoring another one of her essential hormones: testosterone.

Testosterone is important in triggering some of the processes a girl undergoes during puberty.

If testosterone is not at its optimal level, the female body is still a bit out of balance. Since the goal is to truly replace all the hormones to a youthful level, testosterone must be included in the mix.

4) Female Libido Enhancement

One of testosterones primary female functions is helping to control a woman's libido. Research also shows that testosterone levels, which fluctuate dramatically throughout the menstrual cycle, are highest just prior to ovulation. Combine this surge with the influx of progesterone, and it is no wonder that many women feel their greatest sexual drive and energy at this particular time.

Dr. Barbara Sherwin of McGill University in Montreal has studied testosterone replacement in post-menopausal women for the past twenty years. The most dramatic effect she has observed is how testosterone influences a woman's libido. With the decline in hormones at menopause, a woman's sex drive decreases. Some women lose interest in sex altogether.

But Dr. Sherwin's studies show that women who took the testosterone regained their desire for sex and enjoyed it more. These women frequently reported that they experienced more orgasms than before.

86% of post-menopausal women report a decline in their libido and level of sexual activity. Although some part of this change is due to estrogenic deficiency, resulting in vaginal atrophy, loss of energy, and increased depression, most of it is actually caused by a decline in androgens.

The principal areas of testosterone application, depending on the deficiencies being treated, can include the levator ani, the muscle between the pubic bone and the tailbone. This muscle controls the firmness of the vaginal muscle and the muscles that control excretions.

Applications also include differing parts of the female genitalia and other skin-muscle areas for the more generalized testosterone therapy needs. Testosterone placement, and the proper doses, should be specified based on each individual's situation.

In many women, testosterone levels begin falling even before menopause, sometimes resulting in a declining level of sexual interest as early as the late thirties. By the time they reach their forties or fifties many women report a marked sexual decline, sometimes even a feeling of complete sexual deadness.

Overall a woman's level of testosterone declines by approximately 50% in the years after menopause. Perhaps half of this decline is due to the complete shutdown of testosterone production in the ovaries.

Equally important, however, are the adrenal glands declining production of two other important steroids: androstenedione and DHEA. These two hormones have relatively weak androgenic action of their own, but a convenient process converts them to testosterone intra-cellular throughout the body. It is called peripheral conversion.

Those on estrogen HRT complain that the therapy does not bring back the sexual desires and feelings of their youth. This is generally due to a lack of testosterone. Female testosterone levels are frequently lowered by any combination of the following:

Childbirth

Chemotherapy

Surgery (adrenal stress)

Endometriosis

Psychological trauma and depression

Birth control pills

Ovarectomy

Normal aging, including menopause

For a woman to have an optimal sex drive, testosterone levels need to be in the range of 30 to 60 ng/dl.

Testosterone's other effects also have a payoff in terms of sexuality. If a woman has improved muscle tone, more energy, and greater general vitality, this can only enhance her responsiveness once she begins to feel the first stirrings of resurrected sexuality.

As stated, testosterone is also needed by women to help strengthen the levator ani. This muscle controls the firmness of the vaginal muscle and the muscles that control excretions. Many older women lose control of urination and experience leakage as this muscle weakens.

Millions of women begin to suffer bladder leakage in their forties and fifties and don't know what to do about it. Most often they find that when they laugh, cough, or make some intense physical effort, urine escapes. As one patient put it, "Three sneezes and it is time for a change of underwear!"

The reason for the problem is loss of muscle tone in the muscles of the pelvic sling, the levator ani. In both men and women, these muscles are peculiarly dependent on testosterone.

Women who have bladder leakage find that rubbing a small amount of testosterone cream into the area between the bottom of the vagina and the anus will strengthen those muscles, especially if combined with Kegel exercises, an easy to do program that involves periodically contracting the muscles in the pelvic area. Kegel exercises also have a highly favorable effect on sexual function in both women and men.

5) Menopausal Relief

Testosterone does more for a woman than boost her libido. In fact testosterone enhances the functions of estrogen. One of the primary uses of testosterone is for women who take estrogen and progesterone but still have no relief from severe menopausal symptoms.

When these women begin taking testosterone as well, their mood swings and irritability generally disappear.

6) Female Bone Health

As discovered in tests with male testosterone supplementation, testosterone is also instrumental in strengthening the bones and preventing osteoporosis. We have seen that estrogen can slow the destruction of bone but not help rebuild it. Like progesterone, when testosterone is given with estrogen, the damaged bones begin to rebuild and strengthen. So rather than slowing the progression of osteoporosis, optimum hormone therapy can actually reverse it or even prevent it altogether.

7) Decreased Breast Cancer Risk

When women take testosterone in combination with their other hormones, their therapy is much more physiologic than usual. This means that by adding testosterone to the mix, the body better accepts all the other hormones, with fewer side effects and with increased benefits.

One such benefit is a decreased risk of breast cancer in women. Testosterone replacement is essential to a women's overall physical and mental well-being.

8) Benefits of Testosterone HRT and HPT

Testosterone replacement therapies have been practiced for several years. In a test of 94 men in Sweden, 92% of the subjects were able to return to normal; their bodies performed just like men that produced normal levels of testosterone.

In another test, 29 male patients produced notable improvements in erectile functions, libido, and mood within eight weeks.

In another test of thirteen healthy but elderly men, twelve experienced a return to youthful performance.

Many additional tests have been conducted throughout the world. Dr. Perring in London has treated over 800 patients and has shown a return to youthful libido and feelings of well-being and youthful performance when testosterone HRT was taken in conjunction with DHEA.

Collectively, tests over the years have shown that testosterone replacement therapy can achieve the following:

Cause the body to use protein to build:

More and stronger muscles

Thicker skin and improved skin tone

Improved bone density

Decrease the percentage of body fat

Increase strength and endurance

Improved mood

Reverse joint pain

Retard and sometimes reverse osteoporosis

Lower cholesterol

Decrease risk of heart attack

Normalize abnormal electrocardiograms

Lower insulin requirements in diabetics

Improve retinopathy

Eliminate dry skin

Protect against autoimmune diseases

Stimulate growth of certain organs

Regulate production of prostaglandin that keeps prostate growth under control

Nourish urinary and reproduction systems

Stimulate sperm production

Improve libido

Provide better erections

Retard hair loss and grow new and more hair

Stimulate alertness and aggressiveness

Re-activate the telomerase genes to slow aging

Increase life span

Testosterone replacement therapy, HRT, can restore youthful maleness in men and youthful libidos in both sexes. Testosterone precursor therapy, HPT, can approach the effectiveness of HRT but will take longer when safely and effectively used.

9) Testosterone and the Heart

Many practicing physicians have been taught that testosterone causes men to have more heart attacks earlier in life than women. This is a myth that has been proven wrong.

Proof is found by studying the cardiovascular risk factors, which increase as testosterone decreases, like the following:

Cholesterol and triglycerides levels go up, leading to increased arterial plaque

Coronary artery and major artery dilation diminish, hence vasoconstriction and greater risk of cardiac events

Blood pressure rises

Insulin output is increased, which leads to obesity, elevated blood pressure, adult-onset diabetes, and increased cortisone output

Central abdominal fat is increased, leads to increased waist/hip ratio

Estrogen levels are increased, which are associated with higher stroke and heart attack rates

Increased lipoprotein A

Increased fibrinogen, the basis of most blood clots

Decreased human growth hormone (HGH) output, leading to a decline in energy, strength, stamina, and heart muscle mass and output

Decreased energy and strength, causing decreased physical activity, thereby leading to obesity ant the vicious cycle of the male Andropause

Low testosterone levels correlate with more risk factors for heart disease than any other single factor. Testosterone level is far more important to heart disease than cholesterol.

Only a small number of men get heart disease without first showing some of the risk factors listed above, i.e. without first having low testosterone levels.

Testosterone is the heart-protective hormone of the male body, and it can be used to protect men from their major killer: heart disease.

And for men that already have heart disease, testosterone can rescue them from its clutches.

The heart has more testosterone receptors than any other muscle. The heart is the major muscular target for testosterone. The heart's pumping power decreases when testosterone decreases.

Angina pains begin when nitric oxide production declines. Nitric oxide provides a function not unlike Nitroglycerine given to heart patients. Studies show that testosterone stimulates nitric oxide, which not only promotes erectile function in men, for which it is best known, but also promotes cardiovascular health in both sexes.

Nitric oxide is a neurotransmitter that stimulates the nerves causing male erection and vasodilatation, i.e. relaxation and improved blood flow in all major blood vessels, including the Aorta.

In a test conducted by Dr. Shippen on an 80-year-old with heart problems, high blood pressure, angina, and a history of transient ischemic attacks (TIA's), testosterone replacement cured his problems in less than four months. In six months he had resumed significant sex. In three and a half years his cholesterol has gone from 243 to 207 and his HDL from 41 to 55. He has had no further angina or TIAs. At 80!

In a test by Dr. Gerald Phillips at Columbia University College of Physicians and Surgeons, 55 males with chest pain or abnormal stress tests were evaluated. The findings were that the men with higher testosterone had less advanced coronary artery disease and lower risk factors for fibrinogen and Plasminogen (the clot buster), insulin intolerance, and their HDL was higher.

In the Caerphilly Heart Disease study of 2512 men in Wales, it was found that the men with heart disease had lower testosterone, higher insulin, and less HDL.

In a test in China of 62 elderly males with angina, testosterone was given to half and a placebo to the other half. 77% of those receiving testosterone had marked relief from angina compared to 6% for those taking the placebo. This indicates that blood flow to the heart improved 68.8% for those taking testosterone.

In a test by Dr. Shippen, testosterone replacement via a pellet in the buttocks effected the following changes:

At Start of Tests:		5 Months Later
Age:	49	
Height:	5'9	
Weight:	230	220
BP.	192/118	160/100
Cholesterol:	335	235
Triglycerides:	900	357
Blood Sugar:	192	140
Insulin:	70	15
Testosterone:	410	767
Energy:	Always Tired	Energetic
Sex:	Just OK	Very Good
Interest Level	Down	Up

When testosterone levels are low, the risk factors for heart disease are usually high. When testosterone HRT is administered, most of the major risks for heart disease diminish. HPT has a similar effect, although it's not as effective as HRT.

Testosterone replacement is vital for recovery of cardiovascular functions.

10) Testosterone and the Bones

The basic processes of bone build-up and re-absorption were discussed earlier, and it was explained that an osteoblastic stimulator is needed to create a sufficient quantity of Osteoblasts to rebuild the bone lost to re-absorption and other factors.

Testosterone and HGH are nature's best osteoblastic stimulators.

In a test in 1979, a 30-year-old man that suffered severe back pain was found to be in the early stages of osteoporosis. When tested, it was found that his testosterone level was a low 374. After receiving testosterone HRT for only two weeks, his pain ceased. Subsequent tests showed that his new level of testosterone had stimulated his rate of bone mineralization to triple.

Testosterone HRT for men, in some cases, can be far superior to HGH, especially with bone disorders.

Women also frequently need testosterone HRT for certain, actually most, bone disorders. Testosterone can inhibit interleukin-6 (IL-6), which is a hormone-like substance that stimulates the cells in bone marrow. When IL-6 becomes too high, there are more Osteoclasts (the demolition cells previously described) than Osteoblasts. Therefore bone is destroyed faster than it is rebuilt.

So, bone mass and density decrease with age, just as testosterone decreases with age. Testosterone HRT and HPT stimulate the body to re-build bone faster than it is destroyed so that the bone mass and density can return towards their youthful values.

11) Testosterone and Sexual Function

As has been stated, testosterone is the primary sex hormone for men and is the hormone that drives libido in both men and women.

It is very interesting that sexual function and heart conditions in men are closely related. A decrease in sexual function almost always forecasts heart disease and often diabetes.

These are conditions that are common to male Andropause.

Testosterone replacement is vital for restoring libido and sexual function for both males and females.

12) Adverse Side Effects of Testosterone HRT

Un-pure and/or synthetic testosterone can cause many side effects, including liver damage. HRT must use only pure and natural testosterone.

We must also make sure that the nutracuetials used in HPT are of high quality.

Even with pure and natural testosterone there can be adverse side effects, which have been reputed to include an increased risk factor for prostate cancer, atrophying of the testicles, high red blood cell count, depression, fluid retention, reduced sperm count and volume of semen, and a reduction in HDL cholesterol (the good kind).

Of all these concerns, the major concern with testosterone therapy for men has been its potential to stimulate and/or accelerate the growth of benign or malignant prostate tumors. The second major concern has been its reduction of the good HDL, which increases the risk of coronary artery disease.

A series of tests, as described in the next section, and more recent tests reported by Dr. Chein suggest that neither of these concerns is warranted.

According to Dr. Chein, it appears that testosterone HRT has no effect on increasing prostate cancer. His tests show that testosterone replacement therapy lowers both the good and bad cholesterol. It's better to lower both than lower neither.

Dr. Chein has stated that he believes this to be true and that the overall effect of lowering cholesterol with testosterone replacement therapy is an advantage.

Dr. Chein seems certain, but I still have a concern that men susceptible to prostate cancer should be weary of HRT, and if they insist on using testosterone HRT, they should consider individually-tailored dose levels and frequent blood testing.

The third major concern with taking HRT is that the therapy can inhibit the body's own natural production of testosterone. If this happens, the patient must stay on the therapy for the rest of his life.

I believe, as previously stated that HPT is the safer way to increase the availability of testosterone.

HPT avoids this potential problem in that it stimulates the body to use its own natural production system for testosterone.

13) Testosterone and Prostate Cancer

Prostate cancer is the second most fatal cancer in American men (lung cancer is first). About 40,000 men die each year of prostate cancer.

Many physicians were taught, and thus still believe, that prostate cancer is caused by testosterone. The evidence indicates that this is not true.

Dr. A. Moogentaler proved and published his findings in the Journal of the American Medical Association in 1995, stating that prostate cancer is associated with low testosterone.

A study at John Hopkins on fifty men showed no relationship between prostate cancer and testosterone.

Dr. C. W. Lovell treated over 300 men in his Louisiana clinic for a period exceeding thirteen years with testosterone pellets. There was never a single case of prostate cancer.

Dr. George Debled in France reports very low instances of prostate cancers during the twenty years he has given testosterone to more than 2,000 men.

Dr. Shippen in the US reports that his patients with enlarged prostates (BPH) but no cancer all improved when he increased their testosterone levels.

A study in Japan, again of BPH not prostate cancer, showed that the least prostate enlargement correlated with the highest testosterone levels.

Conversely, the Japanese study showed that in the cases where the prostate had become enlarged, such cases were associated with high levels of estrogen.

An American study posed 320 New England men with BPH severe enough for surgery against 320 men without BPH, and it was shown that BPH was more likely in men with low testosterone and high estrogen.

Prostate cancer becomes common in men over the age of 80. Autopsies show that over 30% of men that died from all causes past 80 years of age had prostate cancer.

Fortunately, there are a couple of tests to catch prostate cancer before it becomes life threatening. These two tests are termed PSA and DRE.

When the prostate experiences BPH or cancer, it secretes an antigen termed prostate specific antigen (PSA). Typically:

AGE	PSA
Young	Near 0
Mid-Age	0-4 ng/dl
Problem	
Non-cancer BPH	4-10
Possible Cancer	10+
Most Likely Cancer	20+

This test is fairly accurate, but the DRE exam is highly recommended if the PSA exceeds 4, and is recommended in any case for men over the age of 50. The DRE is a Digital Rectal Exam where the doctor feels the prostate with his finger.

Excessive size will normally prompt a biopsy to test for cancer.

It should also be noted that a good test for indications of prostate cancer might be an analysis of concentrations of testosterone and its more powerful derivative, dihydro-testosterone (DHT). Intriguing support for such a view is offered by several medical studies that show that patients with prostate cancer have lower levels of DHT than patients with normal prostates or with BPH.

The most recent of these, published in the British Journal of Urology, found that the more advanced the cancer the lower the level of DHT. The researchers speculated that a low serum DHT in patients with malignantly transformed glands "may indicate a loss of biochemical differentiation of the tumor."

14) Testosterone to DHT Conversion

Inappropriate testosterone HRT can also cause another kind of problem. The body has two types of an enzyme named 5-Alpha Reductases. There is one in the skin that stimulates oiliness to activate and deactivate hair growth. The second type is mostly in the prostate, and it converts testosterone to a more potent derivative called dihydro testosterone (DHT). DHT is required by the body to perform many functions.

A primary function is to strengthen the fibro muscular portion of the prostate gland. This is vital for male potency and erections. A problem is that too much DHT can cause too much of this growth, resulting in prostate enlargement (BPH) and cancer.

Too much DHT can also cause other problems, like male baldness.

Standard therapy attempts to inhibit the levels of 5-Alpha Reductases so that less DHT is produced. The result frequently causes atrophy of the testosterone-sensitive cells in the stoma, i.e. the fibro muscular portion of the prostate. And this can result in impotency.

15) Testosterone - Estrogen Balance

Young men have testosterone to estrogen rations of 50 to 1. As men get older, these ratios decease to 20 to 1, and they sometimes get as low as 7 to 1.

Too much estrogen in men results in a neutering effect. Too much estrogen can even be more neutering than too little testosterone.

Further, as estrogen increases in men, it causes a slow down in testosterone production, which makes the problem even more severe.

Estrogen begins to occupy the testosterone receptors in the hypothalamus of the brain, tricking it into thinking that it is testosterone. The brain, thinking there is plenty of testosterone, does not order more, and so testosterone levels further decrease.

The man's energy diminishes; sex life falters.

Let's examine what causes this increasing estrogen.

An enzyme called aromatase is widely present in the body and converts a certain portion of testosterone to estrogen. This is a simple process because testosterone and estrogen are chemically quite similar.

This conversion process is necessary for the healthy functioning of estrogen-sensitive tissues in the man's body. Estrogen, for example, is powerfully beneficial to the male brain. Estrogen is vitally necessary for male brain functions.

Too little estrogen will neuter a man just as effectively as too little testosterone.

The window of optimum effectiveness of estrogen in the male body is very small. The control mechanism aspect of estrogen can easily get out of balance as we age. Illness, lifestyles, and more can cause such an out-of-balance situation to occur earlier in life than might otherwise happen.

Such an occurrence may well be the major cause of earlier male Andropause, as previously described. Too much estrogen in the male can cause several harmful effects:

Increased clotting

Narrowing coronary arteries

Increased risk for heart attack

The most common causes of the increases of estrogen in males during their midlife are the following:

Age-related increases in aromatase activity

Alteration in liver function

Zinc deficiency

Obesity

Overuse of alcohol

Drug-induced estrogen imbalance

Ingestion of estrogen-enhancing food or environmental substances

Almost all of these problems are interrelated, and one frequently reinforces or is the outright cause of another. Nonetheless, it's probably useful to take a first look at them separately.

Aromatase activity. First, there is aging itself. As a man grows older, he produces larger quantities of aromatase, the testosterone converter. Consequently he tends to convert higher levels of estrogen. It's possible that being overweight is the main reason for this apparently age-related change. When this is the case, aromatase increase is controllable. When there are other causes, steps to minimize it can be taken.

Liver function. Alterations in liver function involve the important P450 system, a primary processing system that eliminates chemicals, hormones, drugs, and metabolic waste products from the body. Among its many duties is the task of excreting excess estrogen from the body. A wide variety of factors (including alcohol intake) can impair this system and tends to do so with age. In many individuals, this results in a gradual buildup of estrogen. In fact, the P450 system may be the most important factor in metabolic Andropause.

Zinc deficiency. Zinc status is critical. Since Zinc inhibits levels of aromatase, the testosterone-to-estrogen converter, declining zinc will adversely affect the testosterone-to-estrogen ratio. Inadequate levels of zinc are extremely common in the American diet, particularly among the elderly.

In addition, alcohol, drugs, and disease can significantly lower zinc levels. Zinc is also necessary for normal pituitary function, without which the proper hormonal signals will not be sent to the testicles to stimulate the production of testosterone.

There is an interesting circular relationship here. Not only is Zinc important for testosterone, but also testosterone has been found to be necessary to maintain levels of Zinc in the tissues.

Clearly in men whose Zinc status is inadequate, the vicious cycle that becomes established must be broken into at some point through Zinc supplementation.

Obesity. No matter your sex, plumpness tends to estrogenize you. Since fat cells contain aromatase, an increase in fat cell population will cause an increase in testosterone-to-estrogen conversion rate. Moreover, obesity has been clearly associated with lower testosterone levels at all ages. It's not surprising that overweight men almost invariably show signs of an unfavorable testosterone/estrogen ratio.

Alcohol Use. Heavy alcohol intake also causes a dramatic rise in estrogen. Women, for instance, can increase their circulating estrogen levels threefold after just one drink. The rise in men is less dramatic but very significant nonetheless. Alcohol is closely related to two aspects of the problem we just discussed: it inhibits the P450 system, and it decreases Zinc levels.

Heavy drinking in men has long been recognized as causing high estrogen levels with such related symptoms as spider veins, reddish coloration of the palms, gynecomastia (enlarged breasts), and even testicular atrophy. Increased sexual dysfunction is also common.

Shakespeare famously noted, *"Alcohol: increases the desire but decreases the performance."* There is every reason to believe that alcohol-induced estrogen rises are a significant part of that effect.

Drugs. Certain foods, environmental substances, and a variety of prescription drugs have adverse effects. Perhaps the most common class of problem drugs is the diuretics. Millions of American men are taking these water pills to treat high blood pressure.

Though the effects on blood pressure are certainly good in the short term, long-term use of diuretics actually lowers life expectancy. One of the ways it does this is by removing sizable quantities of Zinc from the body. As noted earlier, this increases aromatase, and the long-term estrogen increases that result may cause more cardiovascular damage in men than the diuretics prevent. It is necessary to take fairly high doses of Zinc (50 to 100 mg. daily) to reverse these effects.

Supplemental testosterone HRT can correct unhealthy testosterone to estrogen ratios. It is interesting to compare two of the many tests that have been conducted on this issue.

A 55-year-old man was given testosterone HRT via injections because his testosterone was low. The results:

At Start		A Few Days Later
Testosterone	460	840
Estrogen	20	60

Testosterone shot up to 1200 initially and then stabilized within 24 hours to 840. The estrogen increase from 20 to 60 was far too large a change and could do more damage towards neutering the man than his initial low testosterone would have.

Testosterone injections are always dangerous because they momentarily elevate testosterone too high above natural levels, causing estrogen to go too high. For this reason, most doctors prefer the use of creams and sometimes the patch.

In another test of a 58-year-old man where testosterone was given via a patch, these were the results:

	At Start	A Few Days Later
Testosterone	365	520
Estrogen	52	58

This test also resulted in estrogen at too high a level; however, this man already had his estrogen at too high a level. He was given Zinc and soy protein with the following results:

| Testosterone | 500 |
| Estrogen | 30 |

This is close to the testosterone HRT goals that are practiced by those who are experienced in this field.

16) Atrophy of the Testosterone System

A possible adverse side effect of testosterone HRT is that it may cause the natural system to further shut down. Testosterone HRT providers typically give chorionic ginadotrophin (CG) in conjunction with testosterone to stimulate the system to prevent atrophy.

Those experienced in the field try to avoid this approach as a general practice, reserving its use for special cases that really need it. CG use for most cases is usually counter to the disorder that is causing testosterone to be low in the first place.

There are three commonly recognized endocrine disorders that occur, generally with age, to cause a man to have low testosterone levels. One cause is the male Andropause previously described. The other two are known as primary and secondary hypogonadism. Hypogonadism is a medical term signifying reduced activity of the sexual organs or gonads.

Primary hypogonadism occurs when the Leydig cells in the testicles lose their capacity to secrete testosterone at youthful or near youthful levels.

Secondary hypogonadism occurs when, even if the testicles are capable, the control glands in the brain do not order the testicles to produce.

17) Adverse Side Effects of Testosterone HRT and HPT for Women

Excessive doses of testosterone can cause growth of facial hair, and in extreme cases, a deepening of the voice. Fundamentally, however, there is no justification for a woman ever taking doses high enough to cause such problems. Testosterone is a natural part of a woman's body, and the small supplemental replacement doses normally used by experienced doctors simply brings her back into her normal range, the place where she was from puberty to menopause, the period in which, in all probability, she felt her physical best.

Testosterone therapy for a woman whose levels have been less than ideal is going to stimulate a resurgence of energy, very possibly an improvement in muscle tone, relief from aches and pains, an improvement in bladder problems and in almost all cases, an improvement in sexual desire and energy.

HPT can produce almost all of the benefits of HRT without any of the side effects. It will just not be as quick and effective as HRT.

18 Testosterone Summary

Proper levels of testosterone are necessary for optimum health. The benefits are enormous. There are essentially no adverse side effects of the HPT program. Tests have shown that the proper levels of DHEA is an effective, and when taken properly, safe precursor that will return testosterone levels towards more youthful levels and will, at least partially, re-activate the telomerase genes and slow aging.

Chapter 4.3 Estrogen

Estrogen is the principal female hormone that makes a female a female. The ovaries produce it. Estrogen is the most powerful hormone in the female body. It builds up in young females and peaks shortly after puberty.

Estrogen is also produced and used in the male body. It is vital for brain function, as previously described.

Most all tissues in the human body, over 300, are affected by estrogen. The effects vary from person to person depending on their individual genetic profiles.

After menopause, the female body undergoes major changes because of a significant decrease in estrogen. As an example, the average woman's body at age thirty is 35% fat. By the age of eighty, it is 53% fat.

Estrogen, like testosterone, is an anabolic steroid; though it's anabolic (muscle–building) effect is significantly weaker than testosterone. Its effect on physical shape, on fat deposits around hips and breasts and thighs, is well known. It is also a powerful protector of bone, a guardian of female cardiovascular health, a promoter of thick, smooth skin, and of course, a crucial component in the proper functioning of the female sex organs.

Nothing in medicine has been studied so intensively for so many years and through so many patient trials and investigations than estrogen replacement therapy. Over forty million women have participated in this multibillion-dollar business. Most participants now also use the other key female hormone, progesterone, along with estrogen. Some use progestin, which is a synthetic form of progesterone.

The average woman has almost forty years of life, from puberty to menopause, in which to enjoy the health-promoting benefits of estrogen. During that time she is remarkably resistant to illnesses and to aging changes. A young woman is mankind's healthiest species. Heart attacks and strokes barely exist for women during this part of their lives. Arthritis, and other health problems are rare, and her immune system functions at its best.

And then menopause occurs. The woman loses most of her estrogen, and many things start falling apart.

1) Menopause

Menopause typically begins between the ages of forty-five and fifty-five with the average age being about fifty-one. It is an extreme physical and emotional transition for most women. Menopause is a result of hormonal changes that may occur gradually over several years or suddenly.

The best way to describe the cause of menopause is to start with an understanding of follicle-stimulating hormone (FSH). This hormone, released by the pituitary gland, triggers the growth of follicles in the ovaries. The ovaries, in response, secrete the hormone estrogen.

As menopause approaches, the ovaries become less responsive to FSH, so the pituitary gland produces more in an attempt to maintain estrogen levels. These hormonal changes result in an increasingly irregular menstrual cycle and variable ovulation.

The first sign of menopause for most women is a noticeable change in her menstrual cycle. Bleeding may occur more often or less than it previously had. The length of the menstrual period may become shorter with lighter bleeding or longer with heavier bleeding.

In short, the menstrual period becomes highly unpredictable. The periods may not occur for several months and then reappear. However, about 20% of women will experience no changes in the menstrual cycle until menstruation stops suddenly and completely.

A common symptom of menopause is hot flashes. The secretion of the large amounts of FSH by the pituitary gland causes these. This excessive FSH hormonal imbalance causes the blood vessels in the skin to dilate and constrict irregularly. This then causes the hot flashes and the associated sweating and headaches. About 20% of women do not have hot flashes, but some experience them up to twenty years after menopause!

A very significant result of menopause is a thinning of the vaginal walls. This causes a loss of elasticity and a narrowing of the vagina. It frequently results in dryness with an itching sensation.

Doctors began prescribing various estrogen replacement therapies in the 1940s.

86% of post-menopausal women report a decline in their libido and their level of sexual activity. Although some part of this change is due to estrogenic deficiency resulting in vaginal atrophy, loss of energy, and increased depression, most of it is actually caused by a decline in androgens.

Overall, a woman's level of testosterone typically declines by over 50% in the years after menopause. Half of this decline is due to the complete shutdown of testosterone production in the ovaries.

Equally important, however, are the adrenal glands declining production of two other important steroids: androstenedione and DHEA. These two hormones cannot replace testosterone's contribution to sex drive on their own, but a process in various cells throughout the body converts them to testosterone. It is called peripheral conversion.

The problems caused by menopause are becoming more and more numerous as women continue to live long beyond the onset of menopause. It is estimated that, worldwide, this population of post-menopausal women will increase by 47 million per year!

I should not leave this section on menopause without mentioning "surgical menopause". More than 10 million women in the United States and twice that amount globally have had their ovaries removed for various reasons.

The ever-increasing problems resulting after menopause have to be addressed and treated.

The population of postmenopausal women is rapidly growing worldwide:

1990	467 Million
2030	1,200 Million

2) Estrogen HRT

Estrogen replacement has been offered since the 1950s and is the most widely used of all hormone replacement therapies. However, because of the recent findings on adverse side effects, many women have stopped their HRT, and many others have decided not to start.

The principal fear is that HRT increases the probability of breast cancer. But before we rush to conclusions, let's review the widely varying test data in terms of benefits and adverse side effects.

You will see that HRT is highly beneficial for most women and presents specific, measurable, adverse side effects only for some women.

3) Benefits of Estrogen HRT

Over forty million women in the USA have received estrogen HRT. Most take HRT for the reduction of menopausal symptoms including hot flushes, mood swings, loss of energy, loss of bone density, and loss or reduction of libido. A very large number of researchers have studied various groups of these women at various times and for varying time periods. They have reported a wide range of conflicting results.

In 1999, a panel was convened to reach a consensus on estrogen HRT. They concluded:

Estrogen HRT will decrease the risks of osteoporosis

Estrogen HRT's benefits to the heart are not yet clear

Estrogen HRT may provide increased protection against colon cancer and dementia.

Unfortunately phrases like "not yet clear" and "may provide" are not very useful.

Then in 2002 the very scary results of the Women's Health Initiative were published. The study followed 16,608 women aged 50 to 79 with the average age being 63 at the beginning of the study. The study lasted for a period of 5.2 years. 8,506 of the women were on HRT and 8,102 were given a placebo. The reported findings:

Affect On:	Risk per 10,000 Women
Breast Cancer	Increased 8 more
Heart Disease	Increased 7 more
Stroke	Increased 8 more
Pulmonary embolism	Increased 8 more
Colorectal cancer	Decreased 6 fewer
Hip fracture	Decreased 5 fewer

The scare caused by these results has been greatly exaggerated. Looking closer, it was seen that the women in the 50 to 59 age range – who are the majority of women needing the HRT – enjoyed decreased risks for heart disease and stroke.

Additionally, detailed study of the results indicated that it was the use of synthetic progestin by the women that caused the increased risk of breast cancer. Estrogen in other tests proved to reduce the risk of breast cancer, especially when taken with natural progesterone.

I have carefully analyzed the various tests and studies and taken into account the varying parameters: estrogen alone, estrogen with progestin, estrogen with progesterone, dose size, length of their HRT, the varying genetic profiles and the varying ages of the participants, and I have concluded that the benefits and adverse side effects are dependent on the health and genetic profiles of the individual, and on the combination, balance, and dose size of the HRT hormones.

The combined results from all tests, other than the tests using synthetic progesterone, which should never have been used in the first place, show the following:

A decrease in heart disease that varies from very little for some women up to 60% for others

A decrease in strokes that varies from slight to 75%

Improved mental ability:

Concentration

Alertness

Memory

Retards: Dementia and Alzheimer's disease from slight for some and up to 50% for others

Reduces joint and muscle pain

Retards onset of and sometimes reverses osteoporosis

Keeps bones strong

Keeps teeth strong, 36% less likely to need false teeth

Reduces colon cancer by 29% and up to 55% when used for over 10 years

Provides a slight decrease in risk for lung cancer

When taken with progesterone, the risks of uterine or breast cancer that may result from taking estrogen alone are nullified

Retards onset of cataracts

Increases youthful qualities of skin: thickness and tone

Relief from hot flashes and other symptoms of menopause

Improved mood

Better sleep

More energy

Better quality of life

Longer life, a 44% decrease in mortality over a given period of time

Extends sex life:

Improves libido

Decreases vaginal dryness

Improves vaginal wall thickness

Makes vagina more flexible

Reverses vaginal atrophy

This may seem to be an unbelievable list of benefits, but estrogen is the most powerful hormone in the female body.

Let's look at some more details.

4) Estrogen and the Heart

Many women simply are not aware of the fact that heart disease is the biggest single killer of women as well as men. In fact, all the evidence shows that if it weren't for the protection afforded them by their hormones; women would be significantly more at risk for heart attack and strokes than their male counterparts.

Men have significantly larger arteries, which take a lot longer to get totally blocked. Men are protected to a very large degree by their testosterone, but their protection does not compare with the protection that the female hormones give to women.

Once postmenopausal women lose their hormonal protection, they demonstrate a startling and dismaying ability to overtake the other sex; in less than fifteen years, they're having heart attacks as quickly as men. Yet, in women who replace estrogen, this change does not occur.

The best estimates by reputable medical epidemiologists of estrogen's protective powers are simply stunning. One group of researchers reporting in the New England Journal of Medicine on 5,000 women taking estrogen concluded, based on the improvements in their risk factors, that they would experience a reduction in their rate of heart disease of 42 percent. British researchers, analyzing their own data, came up with a figure of 50 percent.

It is not surprising, for there is hardly a single risk factor for heart disease in women that is not radically improved when a postmenopausal woman replaces estrogen.

Estrogen helps to lower Homocysteine levels and, in combination with vitamin therapy, will almost certainly have a significant life-saving effect.

The meaning of all these alterations in the cardiovascular milieu is best described by looking at each of these factors separately.

Cholesterol: As virtually every American is by now aware, cholesterol has something to do with heart disease. Its importance has been overstressed, but nonetheless, is quite real.

LDL cholesterol, the so-called "bad cholesterol," only causes problems when it has been oxidized by free radicals, the process that antioxidant vitamins like C and E help to protect against.

Once oxidized however, LDL certainly is a bad player. Increased levels of LDL in the bloodstream trigger the activity of macrophages, which are large cells that engulf bacteria and various unwanted debris.

The engorged macrophages then become foam cells, and these trigger changes in the wall of the artery, leading to plaque formation. Plaque then fills up and eventually entirely blocks the artery, the whole process being called atherosclerosis.

HDL cholesterol is called "good cholesterol" because it actually transports LDL out of the tissues and back to the liver for excretion. Estrogen's marked capacity to lower LDL cholesterol and raise HDL cholesterol is an important part of its cardiovascular protection.

Fibrinogen: This natural clot-forming substance in the bloodstream has been associated at high levels with a three-to-five-fold increase in the atherogenicity of LDL cholesterol. High levels of fibrinogen make it far more likely that a blockage in a major artery will result in heart attack. Estrogen is clearly associated with lower fibrinogen levels.

PAI-I: Plasminogen activator inhibitor (PAI-I) decreases the body's ability to inhibit the formation of blood clots and so increases the likelihood that complete blockage of an artery will precipitate a heart attack. Estrogen clearly lowers levels of PAI-I.

Homocysteine: Homocysteine is the newest buzzword in cardiovascular circles.

It derives from metqionine, an essential amino acid that is present at fairly high levels in the American diet. Adequate quantities of vitamins B-6, B-12, and folic acid break down Homocysteine, defusing its potential for harm.

Insulin and Glucose: Both insulin and glucose have been found at higher-than-normal levels to correlate strongly not only with risk of diabetes but also with risk of heart disease. A rise in insulin levels is so common that many doctors regard it as almost a normal part of human aging. Estrogen's tendency to lower these risk factors may be highly significant in the over all cardiovascular protection it offers.

Lipoprotein (a): Levels of lipoprotein (a), a type of cholesterol that has particularly high association with risk for heart attack, seem to be largely determined genetically, but like testosterone, estrogen has turned out to be one of the few things that can effectively lower it.

Results vary from test to test, but it seems very clear that estrogen HRT will reduce heart disease by at least 40%.

These same factors that provide less plaque, better dilating coronaries, decreased clotting factors, and the revving up of the body's natural clot busting system also decrease the probability of strokes. Tests have shown that estrogen HRT will decrease strokes by 75%.

Caution: It should be noted that a very recent test suggests that these cardiovascular benefits of estrogen HRT may not be as great as the previous tests have shown. This latest

test, however, is very suspect because it is counter to the very large number of previous tests, and NIH sponsored it.

Dr. Bruce Ettinger and his associates studied nearly five hundred women who belonged to the Kaiser Permanente health system in California. Two hundred and thirty-two of these women had been on estrogen replacement therapy for an average of seventeen years. They were compared with 222 women who had been on estrogen for an average of less than one year during the same period.

It was discovered that the death rate from all causes for women on estrogen HRT was lowered by 44% over the time period studied.

The American Heart Association has taken the following position: "Since heart disease and stroke kill far more women than any other disease in this country (about one in two women die from cardiovascular disease), the American Heart Association is interested in any research that improves our understanding of how women's risk of cardiovascular disease can be reduced."

The American Heart Association emphasizes the following points:

The analysis report showed that in all women studied, hormone replacement therapy reduced the risk of death from cardiovascular disease, as well as from all causes.

While reduction of risk declined after ten years of treatment, there is still a positive effect, i.e., a reduction in risk continues or persists [even though it is declining] after ten years.

Each woman after menopause should talk with her doctor about what she can do to reduce her risk for cardiovascular disease. This includes: being physically active, following a healthful diet, and not smoking. When the doctor and patient agree, using post-menopausal hormone replacement therapy along with drugs to control elevated cholesterol and high blood pressure have been found to be of great benefit.

Women who take estrogen HRT experience improvement in almost all heart disease risk factors:

Higher levels of "good" HDL cholesterol

Lower levels of "bad" LDL cholesterol

Lower levels of fibrinogen

Lower levels of Plasminogen activator inhibitor (PAI-I)

Lower levels of Homocysteine

Lower levels of insulin

Lower levels of glucose

Lower levels of lipoprotein

Increases blood flow to all parts of the body, including the brain, heart, muscles, skin and bones, and sexual areas.

It is very clear that estrogen HRT, when properly prescribed and in proper combinations with other supplements, will almost certainly provide better heart health for women that have reduced hormone levels.

5) Estrogen and the Brain

Estrogen is vital for brain function. It helps provide the densest possible web of dendrites and axons, the neuronal filaments. These elements connect one brain cell to the next to improve communications. Estrogen accomplishes this by causing the brain cells to be more sensitive to nerve growth factor, a protein whose main function is to stimulate the growth of the dendrites and axons.

Moreover, a fall in estrogen triggers a decrease in blood flow to all parts of the body, including the brain, heart, muscles, skin, and bone. Brain scans of the vascular system of the brain have shown increased circulation when estrogen is added. That means there must be an increase in the delivery of oxygen and essential nutrients. It is difficult to overemphasize how important it is to keep the highways open.

Another benefit of estrogen HRT is its effect on enzymatic changes. Dr. Bruce McEwen, a neurobiologist at Rockefeller University in New York, has shown estrogen spurs the production of choline acetyltransferase, a major enzyme in the brain that is needed to synthesize acetylcholine. Acetylcholine is one of the brain's primary neurotransmitters, a substance that makes possible the final transmission of messages from one brain cell to the next.

People affected with Alzheimer's disease, the most damaging and irreversible of the dementias, have levels of choline acetyltransferase 60 to 90 percent below the human norm. For women, this is caused by a shortage of estrogen. There is no comparable male decline.

The brain is so richly supplied with the aromatase enzyme that by conversion from testosterone, a man's brain is kept richly saturated with estrogen, in sharp contrast with the relative estrogen deprivation a woman's brain experiences once her ovaries have shut down.

Of course, on the male side, this depends on maintenance of adequate testosterone. When testosterone levels in elderly men decline too steeply, either because of natural changes or because of medical treatment that blocks testosterone, brain functions begin to slide downhill quite quickly and consistently.

This finding stimulates the question: "Will administering estrogen HRT to a postmenopausal woman prevent Alzheimer's?"

The answer is maybe, and it is expected to become yes when more tests are completed.

Let's look at some more results.

In one of the more interesting tests of women with Alzheimer's disease, the test subjects experienced some memory return after only three weeks of therapy!

Additional evidence of such improvements comes from a study of 2,418 women over an eleven-year period. The women on estrogen in this test were 40% less likely to get Alzheimer's disease than the women not on estrogen HRT.

In another test, researchers at the University of Southern California studied 235 older women. Eighteen percent of those who had not had estrogen therapy were eventually diagnosed with Alzheimer's disease, compared with only seven percent of the women that had received postmenopausal estrogen replacement therapy.

In another, larger study, Dr. Victor Henderson of the University of Southern California examined the death certificates and medical charts of 2,529 women who had lived in leisure world retirement communities in southern California and who had died between 1981 and 1992. Dr. Henderson discovered that the women who had been on hormone replacement had been forty percent less likely to develop Alzheimer's disease. Moreover, the protection increased with length of use. Women who had taken estrogen for more than seven years were 50 percent less at risk.

A later study in New York City confirmed the pattern.

Doctors at Stanford University gave tests to 72 older women who were estrogen users for an average duration of thirteen years and a control group of 72 women of similar age and education who did not take the hormone. It was discovered that the ability to remember names was 39 percent better among those on HRT.

Dr. Frederick Naftolin, chairman of the department of obstetrics and gynecology at Yale University School of Medicine stated the reason for such great benefits of estrogen HRT: "There is not a cell in the brain that is not estrogen sensitive directly."

Dr. Rowe noted that by the age of eighty, one of six women has contracted Alzheimer's. It appears that estrogen replacement therapy could cut that number in half.

"We know now that women taking estrogen after menopause reduce their chances of getting cognitive impairments."

Dr. John Rowe, President Mt. Sinai School of Medicine New York.

The female body approaches disaster when it loses its most important hormone. Her brain cannot function properly without estrogen. The evidence is overwhelming:

Estrogen stimulates brain function and offers substantial protection against the worst of brain diseases.

6) Estrogen and the Bones

One of the most visible - and catastrophic - results of the lost of estrogen is the subsequent lose of bone. When we see the arms and legs becoming frail and the back beginning to stoop we realize just how important estrogen is to bone health. Let's discuss how this all works.

Osteoclasts are present throughout our lives. They continually break down the bone for it to be reabsorbed into the blood stream. Their counterparts are the Osteoblasts, which continuously build up the bones.

When we are young, the Osteoblasts dominate. During most of our adult lives they are in balance.

Estrogen works by reducing the Osteoclasts, and thereby preventing the increase in bone re-sorption that occurs following the onset of menopause. Estrogen does not seem to have any effect on increasing the rate of bone formation; it just slows its loss.

Progesterone, the other principal female hormone, is a powerful bone-building hormone.

Testosterone is the other hormone that greatly affects bone health. A newer study has shown that the lower a postmenopausal woman's testosterone levels were, the greater her loss of height. This loss is a direct result of bone loss in the spine.

It is now clear that proper HRT with the proper mix of hormones and calcium and other supplements can stop - and in some cases - reverse bone loss.

7) Estrogen and the Skin

The soft, smooth, and attractive skin of a young woman usually changes dramatically after menopause. The wrinkling and coarsening of skin that comes with menopause is largely the result of hormonal changes. Studies show that the condition of a woman's skin depends more on the age at which menopause occurs than on her chronological age. Skin age is determined by how many years a woman goes without adequate estrogen.

Estrogen keeps the layer of subcutaneous fat under the epidermis firm and resilient. Estrogen maintains moisture in the skin by enhancing the production of hyaluronic acid, a substance that keeps water in the tissues. And estrogen maintains the thickness of the skin by supporting the production of collagen, the connective tissue that provides the structure and tone of the skin. When collagen production falls off as a result of estrogen deficiency, a woman's features quickly begin to sag. Reduced collagen, together with the loss of subcutaneous fat, causes tissue to weaken and bruise at the slightest bump.

Researchers at King's College Hospital in London report that skin in women nearing sixty who do not take estrogen is only half as thick as the skin of women who do take estrogen HRT.

8) Estrogen and Sexual Function

Estrogen is the principal female hormone that makes a female a female. Nature created the female primarily to provide children to carry on the species of mankind. She is therefore empowered with one of nature's strongest hormones – estrogen - to enable her to do this.

Estrogen makes a young woman the healthiest member of our species.

Nature did not really design her to live beyond menopause. But advanced hygiene, nutrition, and medicines cause women to live decades and decades after menopause.

After menopause – after the female has given birth to her children and her fertility period is over – nature needs her to live only long enough to raise her last child. Her death after that is not significant to nature. And so our genes had no reason to design her to live longer.

Now women must consider the use of the same knowledge of advanced medicine to restore the hormones that menopause took away.

9) Adverse Side Effects of Estrogen HRT

But there are adverse side effects to HRT, and they differ for each individual.

Early tests conducted in the 1970s indicated that estrogen HRT could increase the risk for breast cancer by 30 to 40 percent when taken for over 5 years. The tests indicated that the risk for ovarian cancer increased 40 percent when estrogen HRT was taken for 6 years and 70 percent when taken over 11 years.

Similar tests reported that HRT also increased the risk of uterine cancer. Other tests indicated a slightly increased risk of venous thrombosis.

Scary.

Later tests in 1980 then showed that these elevated risks are essentially eliminated by the co-administration of progestin, a synthetic form of progesterone. But this combination increased the risk for breast cancer when taken for more than 5 years.

Analysis of the tests also indicated that estrogen HRT decreased the risk of ovarian cancer when taken for less than ten years – but increased the risk when taken over ten years.

The earlier tests of estrogen HRT without progestin showed a significant reduction of the risks for heart disease. But analysis of the later tests after progestin was used with estrogen HRT to nullify uterine cancer risk, it was learned that the progestin had nullified estrogen's benefits for heart disease.

Tests conducted even later show still better results with the co-administration of progesterone rather than it's synthetic.

But then more very scary results from the Women's Health Initiative were published in 2002. See the results as previously presented.

The scare caused by these results has been greatly exaggerated and have led to major confusion. I try to work through the confusion in a later section.

But this confusion has resulted in only 20% of postmenopausal women using any form of estrogen HRT. And of those that do start, 80% quit within three years.

The adverse side effects can usually be prevented for most women by tailoring the correct dose size and hormonal balance.

10) Estrogen and Cancer

Almost all women fear estrogen replacement therapy because of the breast cancer risk. It should be a major concern. Breast cancer is found in 211,000 women in the United States each year. 40,000 die from breast cancer each year. If a woman lives long enough, one out of nine will gets breast cancer in her lifetime.

However, the breast cancer studies that have been conducted for estrogen with progesterone actually show relatively little relationship between estrogen replacement and risk of breast cancer, and many studies report no relationship at all.

The risk of breast cancer is there with or without proper estrogen HRT.

The tests do indicate that some women will increase their risk of breast cancer by taking estrogen HRT. The indications are that risks for these women prone to breast cancer will have their risks increased by 0.15% - that is an increase risk of up to 15 more cases of breast cancer out of 10,000 women.

The increase of risk by 0.15% seems to be a small risk compared with the statistically well-established fact that a woman on hormone replacement therapy is far more likely to live a longer and healthier life than those not taking HRT.

A Kaiser Permanente study done in California over a given period of time in 1996 found that the death rate from all causes was reduced by 44 percent in post-menopausal women who took estrogen HRT.

This study and others like it make it difficult to understand the reasoning of physicians who reject hormone replacement and who even argue that menopause itself does not have a serious negative impact on women's health.

The fact is that the loss of hormones, in both men and women, is part of the process by which nature leads us to old age and death.

It is also interesting to note that when women who are on hormone replacement do get breast cancer, their death rate is markedly lower than it is among breast cancer sufferers who never used hormones. This is because organs such as the breast and prostate stay healthy in the presence of adequate levels of estrogen and testosterone respectively. These hormones cause the typical breast cancers to be less deadly because of a characteristic of normal cells called differentiation.

Differentiation is the processes by which cells that have not yet taken on any particular function, differentiates to do their special assignment, i.e. to become a skin, bone, breast, or any other kind of cell.

Cancer causes the cells that became cancerous to lose differentiation. Cancer takes over cells and converts them to its own purposes, and in the process robs the cells of their functional nature. Eventually the cancer cells lose all functional resemblance to other cells in the organ or tissue where they're found.

But in postmenopausal women on estrogen replacement who do contract breast cancer, their cancer cells are different. The cells remain much closer to the normal type of breast cell than do the cancer cells of women not on estrogen HRT. As a result, the tumor is generally less advanced and tends not to grow as swiftly and aggressively as does a normal cancer cell.

Estrogen's processes of differentiation serves the women well because the differentiation process prevents the cancerous cells from becoming as severe as they otherwise would.

As for colon cancer, tests have shown that estrogen therapy will reduce this cancer by 29%. When estrogen was taken over a ten-year period, the reduction increased to 55%.

It should be noted however, that even if the risks of cancer of the uterus were not increased, estrogen HRT would most likely cause a slight increase in benign fibroid tumors in the uterus. It is also likely to slightly increase the risks for blood clots, gallstones, migraine headaches, breast tenderness, and weight gain.

Studies show however that the probabilities of these adverse side effects occurring for an individual are less than one percent.

11) Adverse Side Effects of Estrogen: Summary

The more conservative position is that estrogen HRT – even with progesterone – may slightly increase the risk of breast cancer. It may also increase the risk for ovarian and uterus cancer.

Even if the risks of cancer of the uterus are not increased, estrogen HRT will most likely cause a slight increase in benign fibroid tumors in the uterus. It is also likely to slightly increase the risks for blood clots, gallstones, migraine headaches, breast tenderness, and weight gain.

There are unresolved questions on estrogen's effect on strokes.

Such risks can be essentially eliminated by using HPT instead of HRT.

Chapter 4.4 Progesterone

While estrogen is the primary female hormone – the secondary female hormone, progesterone, is vital for principal female functions. It is also produced primarily in the ovaries. Progesterone begins to be produced at the beginning of puberty and then cycles monthly. It declines to less than 10% of its peak after menopause.

Progesterone causes the lining of the uterus to thicken in preparation for pregnancy, and when pregnancy occurs, is essential for normal functioning and the healthy development of the baby. At the end of pregnancy, a fall in the level of progesterone helps initiate labor.

But progesterone should not just be considered a female hormone. It is not a sex hormone; it plays no part in the secondary sexual characteristics, which develop at puberty.

It plays a major role in the bodies of both men and women. Progesterone levels should be optimized to maintain good health. Levels vary considerably in women, rarely in men.

Progesterone is the precursor to the two sex hormones: estrogen and testosterone.

It is secreted primarily by the ovaries in females and the testes in men. Smaller amounts are produced by the adrenal glands, the brain and glial (nerve) cells.

There are no great quantitative differences between men and women except in a woman's latter phase of the menstrual cycle. It's in this last phase of the monthly cycle that progesterone levels rise considerably above that found in the first half or follicular phase. It rises from as little as less than 1 ng/mL to 20 ng/mL.

It is the fluctuating progesterone levels, together with the rise and fall of estrogen, that result in changes of mood, sleep patterns, cravings/appetite, PMS, etc.

It is the ratio between estrogen and progesterone that causes problems. If there is too much estrogen in relation to progesterone then the problems become more severe.

Estrogen is an excitatory hormone, causing cells to divide and multiply, including fat cells. It's implicated in inflammation, cancer, endometriosis, fibroids, PMS, migraines/headaches, cravings, incontinence, generalized aches and pains, flaking nails and weight gain.

Progesterone, on the other hand, is a calming hormone, reversing or preventing the above symptoms.

Progesterone and estrogen are the two hormones currently given in HRT for postmenopausal women. Originally estrogen was replaced alone, but doctors discovered this increased the risk of uterine cancer, and so progesterone was added.

Recently a major test was terminated because it showed that the combination of estrogen and a synthetic version of progesterone caused an increase in some adverse side effects, as are described above in the Estrogen Section.

1) Progesterone and Cancer:

Early studies of women on estrogen HRT indicated that it increased not only the risk for uterine cancer, but it also increased the risk for breast cancer. Doctors therefore began to switch from estrogen alone to a combination of estrogen and progestrogestin, a synthetic form of progesterone.

Provera is a synthetic form of progesterone that was and is widely used. The synthetics were used because Progesterone had been too expensive.

Natural progesterone is now available at affordable prices, and therefore most medical professionals recommend against use any of the synthetics.

2) Synthetic Progesterone

A good reason not to use synthetics progesterone is demonstrated by the following typical case of a woman on Provera. She was fifty-eight, and she was miserable for the five or six years after menopause.

Her body felt sore, and her brain felt battered from a long battle with her nerves. Her sex life had shriveled. She had retired at fifty-five, thinking that maybe with more time and less work all would improve. And nothing had.

She had acute anxiety, periodically acute depression, and was subject to panic attacks. All her problems had started at her change of life. There were mostly vaguely psychiatric. She had tried a wide variety of anti-anxiety and antidepressant drugs with little effect but plenty of side effects. She summed up her feelings: "I feel my life is totally out of control, and there's absolutely noting I can do about it."

And yet, what seemed mental was purely hormonal. As soon as she switched from Provera, the synthetic progesterone she was taking, to natural progesterone, and started applying a modest amount of testosterone cream daily, her mental problems vanished, and her original talkative, bubbly personality emerged. Her sex drive came back; her energy soared.

Some of her depression had no doubt been due to the synthetic progesterone, which affects many women that way, but the other effects were almost certainly the result of putting androgens back into a deprive body. Tests have shown that her ovaries were totally shut down, and her adrenal glands were producing virtually no DHEA or testosterone.

The use of progesterone with estrogen HRT provides all the benefits of estrogen HRT and nullifies the potential increased risk for cancer.

The use of pure progesterone as opposed to use of one of its less costly synthetics will prevent the side effects that some women have to the synthetics.

There is however still a concern that estrogen-progesterone HRT can produce adverse side effects if used for 4 years or more. These concerns can be minimized by taking the proper doses tailored for the individual, alternated with Hormone Precursor Therapy, and closely monitored for any adverse side effects.

3) Progesterone and the Bones

Estrogen prevents the increase in bone re-sorption that occurs following the onset of menopause. Estrogen appears, however, to have no effect on increasing the rate of bone formation, which means it's important to set it in place as a sort of metabolic shield against osteoporosis before the ravages of bone loss occur.

In contrast to the effects of estrogen, a great deal of evidence now suggests that progesterone, its partner in the management of the female reproductive cycle, is a powerful bone-building hormone. In effect, this means that two out of three post-menopausal women who still have an intact uterus, and who should be taking progesterone and estrogen to protect themselves from the greater risk of uterine cancer that estrogen replacement alone may cause, are actually lucky. The progesterone they take will not only negate (and, according to some studies, even reduce) any increased risk of cancer, but it will also add a powerful building block to their plan for bone preservation.

4) Adverse Side Effects of Progesterone HRT

There are no known adverse side effects of progesterone at any dosage. This is because overdoses do not suppress the body's own production. This is because progesterone stimulates for its own synthesis.

Chapter 4.5 DHEA (Dehydroepiandrosterone)

DHEA is a hormone produced primarily by the adrenal glands from cholesterol. It is called the Mother Hormone because it is converted by the body on demand into other hormones, including the following;

Estrogen

Progesterone

Testosterone

Androstenedione

About half of the body's DHEA is produced in the adrenal cortex, with the rest coming from gonads, fat tissue, and the brain. The steroid synthesis pathway is Cholesterol > Pregnenolone > DHEA > testosterone > estrogen.

DHEA is also the Mother Hormone because it provides great health and longevity benefits. It begins to be produced by the male at the age of seven, increases to its peak at about age twenty-five, and decreases to near zero in old age as depicted in the previous chart.

Female production is less than the male and peaks near age twelve and decreases with age as also depicted in the chart.

DHEA is a hormone precursor produced naturally in the adrenals, brain, and gonads. The decline of DHEA production with age results in low serum DHEA that contributes to many age-related degenerative diseases.

DHEA is a master hormone metabolized in the adrenals to make other hormones. Supplementing with DHEA has been shown to increase energy levels, vitality, and a sense of well-being

Nearly every cell in the body has receptor sites for this unique hormone. DHEA levels in the blood can indicate the present and future status of certain diseases, including the following:

Cancer

Immune system functions

Cardiovascular disease

Memory disorders

Aging status

The DHEA levels in an individual are the best hormonal indication of how that person is aging. The slower one loses their DHEA as they grow older, the slower they age.

1) Benefits of DHEA HRT and HPT

A very large number of tests conducted by many researchers over a long period of time have shown that DHEA can provide the following benefits:

Enhance the immune system, stimulating T-cell production that fights invading germs and producing protection against the following:

Cancer

Atherosclerotic

Osteoporosis

Lupus

Herpes

Hepatitis B

Influenza

Diphtheria

Tetanus

Adds neurons to the brain that helps with the following:

Improves memory

Helps with learning disorders

Retards Alzheimer's disease

Helps with weight control by doing the following:

Raises Metabolism

Decreases Appetite

Decreases fat storage

Converts fat to lean muscle

Provides youthful Health

Prolongs Life

DHEA has been shown to prolong life by preventing and/or controlling or curing many of the diseases associated with aging. It enhances the immune system and protects against the diseases listed above.

It lowers blood cholesterol and stabilizes blood sugar levels. It assists in weight loss and in the conversion of fat to lean muscle mass.

It deserves being called The Mother of all Hormones.

In a test by endocrinologist Samuel Yen, DHEA increased muscle in both men and women, and the men gained strength and lost fat. But the most noticeable effect was the way the drug made people feel.

In a previous study of thirty middle-aged people, Yen found that 82% of women and 67% of men scored higher on a series of tests measuring their ability to handle stress, their quality of sleep, and overall well-being when they were on DHEA.

Dr. Regelson, a leading oncologist states: "If you want to maintain a youthful level of health, then you have to be youthful physiologically and that means maintaining youthful levels of these (DHEA) hormones."

DHEA wakes up elderly immune systems and restores them to youthful levels of efficiency.

Dr. Daynes of Utah mixed DHEA with his vaccines and showed a great improvement against hepatitis B, Influenza, Diphtheria, and Tetanus, and he also reported that DHEA stimulates T-cell proliferation to fight invading germs.

And studies have shown DHEA to work against obesity by raising metabolism, decreasing appetite, and decreasing fat storage. It decreases fat storage by blocking the glucose - 6- phosphate – dehydrogenises enzymes (G 6 p D). That blocks the body's ability to store and produce fat.

DHEA decreases appetite by stimulating the body to produce cholecy to kinin (CCK), the substance that signals our brain that we are "full."

In a study in 1988, five normal men of normal weight were given a dose of 1600 mg of DHEA per day for twenty-eight days. Their average body fat was decreased by 31% and replaced with the exact same weight in lean muscle. Their LDL dropped by 7.5%, thus protecting against cardiovascular disease.

Replacing our youthful levels of DHEA positively affects each and all of these effects of aging. DHEA can prevent and/or help cure many of the diseases of aging. DHEA can make us younger.

2) Adverse Side Effects of DHEA HRT

But a word of caution: High doses of DHEA will suppress the body's natural ability to produce DHEA. If one allows this to happen, then one has to continue to take DHEA for the rest of their lives.

Too much DHEA can also act as an oxidant to disrupt normal cell function. These concerns can be avoided by taking the proper dose levels and by supplementing it with the proper levels of antioxidants.

Experts in the field generally limit the daily doses to between 25 and 150 mg (as compared to the 1600 mg given in the 1988 study previously discussed). The precise level is individualized for each patient by detail blood and other analysis. Further, the daily doses are broken down into at least 2 doses per day to minimize DHEA levels.

And the DHEA is always given as part of the antioxidant, enzyme, and hormone mix tailored to each individual.

Chapter 4.6 Melatonin

Melatonin is a natural hormone that exists in all living creatures. It was discovered in 1958. It is produced by the pineal gland from the amino acid Tryptophan and was earlier determined to be secreted by the pineal gland in our brain. We now know that it is also secreted by other endocrine glands as described below.

Melatonin is the most powerful regulator of the body's biological clock and the immune system. It has been termed The Wonder Drug.

1) Melatonin as the Biological Clock

That portion of Melatonin that regulates our biological clock is secreted by our Third eye, the pineal gland located near the center of the brain, between the eyes. In some of the more primitive animals – such as reptiles – it is literally a third eye in that it is a light-sensitive organ covered by a shield of clear cartilage.

The pineal gland helps govern circadian rhythms, i.e. our biological rhythms that take place over a 24-hour day. In more primitive animals, it also governs seasonal cycles of mating, migration, and hibernation.

Tests have shown that when people spend fourteen hours or more a day in darkness that they return to primordial sleep patterns, during which they produce the high levels of Melatonin our ancestors experienced and the return to the natural pattern of restful sleep.

But the levels of Melatonin decline as we age. As they decline, we get sleep problems such as insomnia. A Gallup survey reports that 49%

of American adults, mostly older adults, suffer from insomnia.

Dr. Steve Novil of the American longevity Research Institute has been treating patients with Melatonin since 1990, and their insomnia has been cured.

Studies and tests by The University of Surrey in Britain, and by French researchers have shown that Melatonin can be used to reset our internal clocks as a cure for jetlag by taking 8 mg of Melatonin on the day of the flight and for three days thereafter; the test subjects were able to sleep better, focus better, and experienced fewer mood swings then did the control group that took a placebo rather than Melatonin.

2) Benefits of Melatonin HRT

But Melatonin is much more than a substitute sleeping pill. Its benefits include:

Cure for insomnia

Resets "clock" from travel

Lethal to some cancers:

Melanomas

Breast

Prostate

Inhibits others (but this is less proven)

Protects against chemotherapy-induced toxicity

Protects against a variety of degenerative and age-related neurological conditions of the brain:

Parkinson's disease

Alzheimer's disease

Schizophrenia

Depression

Protects against other diseases:

Diabetes

Asthma

Down's Syndrome

possibly AIDs

Protects against cataracts

Lowers cholesterol

Increases sexual interest

Grows sexual organs back to youthful sizes

Keeps thymus gland active into old age, further improving immune system

The very best antioxidant to fight free radicals

Increases lifespan

Restores youth

Dr. Walter Pierpaoli was the first to show that Melatonin treatments can extend the life span of mice by 25%. Others have increased this to 200%. These experiments were verified and extended by Dr. Pierpaoli working with Russian Dr. Lesikov. They transplanted the pineal glands from old mice to young mice and vice versa. The old mice lived out the longer remaining lifespans of the young mice and vice versa.

Converting mouse life to human life suggests that Melatonin treatments alone could increase human life span to 150 years. (Or at least 120 years – to the limits caused by telomere erosion previously discussed.)

One of the principal reasons Melatonin can extend life is that it is the very best natural scavenger of free radicals. It is nature's best antioxidant. It removes the free radicals (oxidants) from our cells. Otherwise they will cause cell damage and even DNA damage.

Studies have shown that Melatonin is a more powerful antioxidant than vitamins E and C for acting as a free radical scavenger and for protection against aging. Melatonin is also more efficient than vitamin E as a scavenger of the peroxyl radical, which contributes to massive lipid destruction in cell membranes.

Melatonin also protects against a variety of degenerative and age-related neurological conditions of the brain, such as Parkinson's disease, Alzheimer's disease, schizophrenia, and depression. Melatonin has also been shown to prevent cataracts.

Melatonin enhances the immune system and has been found to have a powerful inhibitory effect on some cancer cells. Further, Melatonin has been shown to amplify immune effects of interleukin-2 and to protect against chemotherapy-induced toxicity. In tissue cultures, Melatonin has direct lethal action on melanoma cancer cells and estrogen-sensitive breast cancer cells. Melatonin has also been found to inhibit prostatic cancer cells from proliferation.

Also related to immunity is the research that has shown the dramatic effect of Melatonin on the thymus gland. The thymus gland is important in the defense against infection. The thymus gland undergoes a transformation as we age. The thymus gland grows steadily larger as we approach puberty, and then it begins to shrink until; in old age, it has virtually disappeared. As the thymus declines, so does our infection-fighting ability. Melatonin appears to protect this gland and improve its function as we grow older.

Tests have also shown that Melatonin may be effective in treating diabetes, asthma, cataracts, Down's syndrome, breast cancer, and even AIDS.

It appears to help with other cancers. Doctors in Milan added Melatonin to their chemotherapy and immunotherapy and got significant tumor reductions that enabled their cancer patients to live longer.

It was most effective in treatment of breast cancer, where it almost always retarded it and frequently cured it. Early tests indicate that it may be equally effective against prostate cancer – a cancer chemically related to breast cancer.

It also lowers cholesterol in those who have high cholesterol, thereby helping to prevent heart disease. It does not appear to affect cholesterol when cholesterol is at a normal level.

These tests results suggest that Melatonin has evolved to become a much more versatile hormone for humans than it is in more primitive animals.

Dr. Pierpaoli believes that Melatonin has evolved to become the principal messenger that tells our bodies when to enter puberty, begin sexual development, start each menstrual cycle in females, put us to sleep, wake us up, and when to produce antibodies to combat disease.

Dr. Klatz has likened the pineal gland to the orchestra conductor that uses Melatonin as a kind of baton.

It appears that as we evolved and Melatonin took on all these messenger functions, it also began to be produced in glands in addition to the pineal gland. Very recent studies have shown that Melatonin is also produced in the retina – which acts as a photo-protectant to light sensitivity in the eye. This probably evolved as our third eye, the pineal gland, regressed back into the brain, and could no longer directly sense light

The very recent studies have also shown that Melatonin is produced in the endocrine cells that live in the gut. In fact, it seems that the gut now produces more Melatonin than the pineal gland.

I speculate that as Melatonin took on ever increasing roles as messengers to various organs those glands closer to the source of messenger developed. Thus the gut produces its own Melatonin as a messenger to the thymus.

Melatonin stimulates the thymus to release the T-cells that fight invading germs.

Melatonin treatments have also rejuvenated patients' sexual interest, and in several cases, have caused sex organs to grow back to their youthful sizes.

In summary, Melatonin restores youth.

3) Future Benefits of Melatonin HRT

Melatonin is now being studied to develop treatments for (1) stress, (2) improving immune system, (3) helping with mental disorders, and (4) as an ingredient in a new birth control pill.

4) Adverse Side Effects of Melatonin HRT

All tests have shown that Melatonin is completely harmless to the body at all dose levels. High doses, however, can cause a natural drowsiness and therefore should be taken only at bedtime.

Experts in the field limit the amount and timing of Melatonin treatments. Proper doses simulate the amount and release cycles of the youthful body. Proper Melatonin therapy always uses Melatonin only in conjunction with the other elements of the enzyme/hormone mix.

Chapter 4.7 Pregnenolone

Pregnenolone hormone is a steroid precursor produced in the brain and in the Adrenal gland. It is a precursor for DHEA and progesterone hormones – which are produced from Pregnenolone based on the body's need. DHEA and progesterone are then precursors for the specialized steroid hormones:

Cortisol

Aldosterone

Estrogen

Testosterone

"Of all the hormones in the body, the precursor hormone, Pregnenolone, may be the most important for health and longevity." D. Gary Young

"If DHEA is the mother hormone, Pregnenolone is the grandmother, because it is the precursor to DHEA." Dr. Chein

1) Early History

But most people have not heard about Pregnenolone and its amazing benefits. One reason has to do with drug companies and profits.

Pregnenolone research in the early 1940s was very promising and showed that Pregnenolone is effective in relieving arthritis pain, reducing PMS and menopausal symptoms, fighting stress and fatigue, improving memory, and lifting mood. But just as this research was being printed in medical journals, the discovery of synthetic cortisone was announced.

Drug companies could patent their laboratory version of cortisone and then make huge profits.

Pregnenolone, however, is a natural substance and is not patentable. Because synthetic cortisone was so fast-acting and offered great profit potential, Pregnenolone research was basically abandoned.

It was not discovered until later that cortisone had terrifying side effects (immune system suppression and osteoporosis being the two most devastating).

Pregnenolone has been shown to be virtually free of side effects.

A man in one Pregnenolone study did develop a temporary rash; in another study on memory, a participant reported the side effect of decreased symptoms of arthritis! Sounds like a good side effect to me!

2) Pregnenolone and Arthritis

The beneficial effects of Pregnenolone on arthritis and other bone, joint, and muscle diseases are well documented. In two studies on ankylosing spondylitis, an inflammatory disease of the joints that causes back pain and stiffening, patients showed marked improvement when treated with Pregnenolone.

Tests have also shown it to be anti-inflammation. It was widely used to treat rheumatoid arthritis until the discovery of the more effective cortisone that is now used for this disease. It is still used for patients that cannot tolerate cortisone's adverse side effects.

Neurobiologist Dr. Eugene Roberts studied the arthritis research from the 1940s and 1950s and said: "Treatment with PREG (Pregnenolone) can be maintained indefinitely without apparent harmful effects and is much less expensive than with ACTH or cortisone or with other anti-inflammatory steroids."

In addition Pregnenolone provides other significant biological functions throughout the body and provides the benefits described below.

3) Pregnenolone and Memory

Pregnenolone has long been known as a memory hormone.

In a recent study Drs. John E. Morley, James F. Flood, and researcher Eugene Roberts studied the effects of several hormones on the learning and memory abilities of rats. Researchers taught the rats the route through a maze. Then the rats were given DHEA, Pregnenolone, or testosterone.

To test the effect of the hormones on memory, the rats ran the maze again one week later. The Pregnenolone-treated rats greatly outperformed even those that were given the other hormones, and this performance was achieved using unbelievably small doses of Pregnenolone.

Research on memory by Rahmawhati Sih, Ph.D. showed that after older men and women were given Pregnenolone, the memory tests given three hours later showed gender variation. The women rated higher in verbal recall, while men improved in visual spatial tasks that required three-dimensional thinking.

The dramatic results of this test and the earlier human tests from the 1940s earned Pregnenolone the title of most powerful memory enhancer, up to 100 times more powerful than other hormones.

4) Pregnenolone and Alzheimer's disease

Positive discoveries have led to current studies, including several currently evaluating the potential of Pregnenolone to treat Alzheimer's disease. Many people believe Pregnenolone could be effective in treating even full-blown Alzheimer's disease because studies have shown that Alzheimer's patients have much lower levels of the hormone than healthy individuals of a similar age. Pregnenolone may also aid in Alzheimer's treatment because it is a precursor to estrogen and progesterone, which, in recent years have been shown to help prevent the onset of this terrible disease.

5) Benefits of Pregnenolone HRT

Tests have also resulted in Pregnenolone being recommended for all diabetics over the age of 40 and sometimes even younger diabetics.

Pregnenolone can also be a great help for easing the trauma of menopause. This is especially true for the dreaded ordeal for the millions of women who choose not to use estrogen replacement therapy because of a four to eight times higher chance of uterine cancer.

Part of the reason Pregnenolone has such a powerful effect on so many areas of the body is its grandmotherly role. As Pregnenolone levels increase, typically so will those of DHEA and the sex hormones of which it is a precursor. This is part of what allows Pregnenolone to improve overall physical and mental health.

Recent studies have shown that male and female bodies use Pregnenolone differently. Given the same amounts of the hormone and the same tests, results vary by gender. The conclusion from these studies is that in women, more of the Pregnenolone becomes estrogen, while men use more Pregnenolone to make testosterone.

As the parent hormone from which all other vital steroid hormones are made, Pregnenolone has been intensively studied for its effects on health, longevity, and emotional well-being.

Pregnenolone is made from cholesterol in the body. In turn, it can be synthesized into a number of hormones: estrogen, progesterone, testosterone, DHEA, Aldosterone, cortisol, etc. It is, in fact, the master hormone from which all the steroid hormones are derived.

A rising tide of clinical research is just beginning to show the powerful therapeutic benefits of natural Pregnenolone. Benefits that can reverse decline, balance hormones, and increase longevity. All in a completely natural substance that is non-toxic and virtually without side effects!

You can rest assured that Pregnenolone is well tolerated, and its safety has been well documented. William Regelson, M. D. and Carol Colman stated in their book, The Super-Hormone Promise: Nature's Antidote to Aging, "We know that Pregnenolone is safe, well tolerated, and causes no know side effects.

6) Some Concerns

The body needs the following components to produce adequate amounts of Pregnenolone:

Cholesterol

Thyroid hormone

Certain enzymes

Vitamin A

If levels of these components are insufficient, the Pregnenolone supply will be too low. This can result in obesity, memory impairment, and aging-related disorders.

7) Lack of Cholesterol Hurts Pregnenolone Levels

Now scientists and researchers are again looking at the value of Pregnenolone. The research that D. Gary Young found establishes how Pregnenolone declines in the body more than 60 percent between the ages of 35 and 75. Along with this natural bodily decline, our bodies have had to deal with a decrease in the building block of Pregnenolone – cholesterol. "Low cholesterol" or "no cholesterol" has been pounded into the heads of health-conscious consumers.

While the cholesterol link to heart disease is under question today, cholesterol-lowering drugs are causing hormone imbalance. Without cholesterol, there is no Pregnenolone, which means the body cannot create the hormones it needs.

The lack of cholesterol (and thus Pregnenolone) in our diets may be the cause of many cases of depression. Dr. William Regelson writes that: "A recent study conducted by the National Institutes of Mental Health showed that people with clinical depression have lower than normal amounts of Pregnenolone in their cerebral spinal fluid (the fluid that bathes the brain)."

Spinal cord injuries may be minimized with Pregnenolone according to a number of rat studies. Dr. Eugene Roberts would like to see a Pregnenolone cream placed in first aid kits for use on the spine following earthquakes or accidents.

He explained the value of the Raindrop Technique where certain oils are dropped along the spine: "Along the spine happens to be one of the largest accumulations of receptor nerve sites, and that's why Raindrop Technique works so specifically. When the oils get in there and can start stimulating nerve transmission – that's very, very important. When you combine the oils with Pregnenolone, then the oils carry the Pregnenolone into the cell structure to start that cell's rejuvenation. It is win, win, win, and balance, balance, balance."

Men are also susceptible to the age-related loss of Pregnenolone in the body. They needn't fear that Pregnenolone might be turned into a female hormone.

8) Adverse Side Effects of Pregnenolone HRT

There are no known adverse side effects at any dosage. This is because overdoses do not suppress the body's own production. This is because Pregnenolone stimulates for its own synthesis.

So while Pregnenolone treatments per se appear to be completely safe, we need to monitor all the hormones to make sure that the use of Pregnenolone, acting as a precursor for other hormones, does not adversely affect them.

I have already shown that too much DHEA, estrogen, or testosterone in the body can cause some unpleasant side effects. When your physician carefully monitors not only your Pregnenolone levels but also all your hormone levels, you can safely enjoy the benefits of Pregnenolone including increased mental acuity, better memory, and a greater sense of well-being.

Chapter 4.8 Thymus Hormones

The thymus gland, which is located in the thorax behind the sternum (chest bone), secretes thymus hormones. It is the primary lymphatic tissue that secretes thymus hormones. Its function is to secrete hormones to nurture lymphocytes.

There are two types of lymphocytes: killer cells that destroy foreign substances, i.e. bacteria, viruses, cancer cells, and other foreign bodies that are not a natural part of the healthy, body and helper cells that locate and mark the foreign substances for the killer cells.

The thymus provides at least six types of cells:

Interleukin 1, which is a class of proteins that are secreted mostly by macrophages and T cells.

Interleukin 2 is another version of the Interleukin proteins.

Interleukin 6 is yet another version of the Interleukin proteins.

Thymosin is a hormone that influences the development and differentiation of T-cells.

Thymopoietin, with the formal name of thymin, is any one of three polypeptide hormones that result by alternative splicing of the same gene.

Thymulin is a zinc-dependent thymic hormone that regulates the differentiation of the immature thymocyte (precursor of a T cell) subpopulation and the function of mature T and natural killer cells.

The combination of the last 3 items is known as thymic humoral factor (THF), and it is frequently used in HRT in place of the full set of thymus hormones.

The thymus gland is large at birth. It atrophies a great deal by age twenty.

The thymus hormone level builds to a peak at puberty and goes to less than 20% of its peak by age twenty. It then continues to decrease linearly to less than l0% of its peak by age eighty.

The thymus gland is the major part of our immune system. In childhood this gland helps develop our immune system, with its principal task being the creation of T-lymphocytes, the specialized cells that find helper cell lymphocytes and eliminate bacteria, viruses, and foreign matter from the body. In late childhood, the thymus is the size of a plum, but at puberty it begins to shrink, and by the time we reach old age it is no larger than a small raisin.

Some of the functions of the thymus get transferred to other areas of the body such as the lymph nodes and bone marrow, but the atrophication of the thymus has a well-defined relation to immune system decline.

According to the statisticians, a human being is least likely to die of disease at the age of twelve, when his or her thymus is in full flower, than at any other time in life.

We now have considerable evidence in animals and some indications in humans that

HGH could regenerate the thymus. Research in the 1980's on dogs showed that when growth hormones were inserted, "the thymuses of growth hormone-treated dogs regenerated, and resembled the thymic tissue of young dogs."

In 1991 David Khansari and Thomas Gustad of North Dakota State University completed a long-term study on mice. Taking fifty-two mice that had reached the age of senescence (approximately seventeen months); they divided them into two equal sized groups with one group receiving growth hormone for thirteen weeks. Most of the members of that group were still living after all members of the control group had died.

Thymus function provides for the development of:

The killer and helper lymphocytes

The central nervous system

The pituitary gland in the brain

The operative word for the thymus gland is development. When a person's development is complete – by age twenty or there about – the gland's secretions decrease to the point that we cease to develop, and we then begin to age.

The deterioration of the thymus gland is closely linked to learning and memory abilities; and to the age-related diseases.

All six of the hormones that are secreted by the thymus gland are found to have an effect on T-lymphocyte differentiation and activation. The three hormones that make up the thymic humoral factor, i.e. Thymosin, Thymulin, and Thymopoietin inter blood circulation and act on the lymphocytes and tissues at various sites in the body.

1) Benefits of Thymus HRT

Research has identified the dependence of the central nervous system's development on thymus gland function. Other studies have established an important interaction between the thymus gland and the development of the pituitary gland in the brain. The age-related deterioration of learning and memory abilities has also been linked to the atrophy of the thymus gland.

In addition to the central nervous system, the thymus gland may also affect functions of other endocrine tissues. For example, congenital absence of the thymus gland is associated with alterations of the pituitary gland, adrenal gland, thyroid, and ovaries.

Anti-thyroid drugs that induce hypothyroidism also cause a marked atrophy of the thymus gland.

T-4 is one type of thyroid hormone. When its levels were reduced following anti-thyroid medication treatment, the thymocyte population in the thymus gland was also reduced. Conversely, when T-3, a different type of thyroid hormone, was administered in mice, multi-facilitated effects included increased weight and cell population as well as enhanced thymocyte production.

Within thirty days after surgery, removal of the pituitary gland resulted in a 50% reduction in both thymus gland weight and concentration of the thymus hormone known as Thymosin.

Over the past twenty years, at least four separate and distinct thymus preparations have been isolated and analyzed for T-lymphocyte regulating properties. Thymosin, Thymulin, Thymopoietin, and thymic humoral factor (THF) have been utilized as thymic hormonal preparations for hormone replacement therapy. Thymosin (TF) is a group of low molecular weight proteins extracted from bovine thymus.

Thymosin has displayed potent stimulatory effects on T-lymphocyte-mediated immunity. Thymosin increases lymphocyte activity and enhanced IL-6 production in spleen cells. Thymosin had a stimulating effect on luteinizing hormone and genadotropin releasing hormone, both pituitary hormones, in vivo studies of pituitary tissues.

In vitro Thymosin studies show that another pituitary hormone known as prolactin is released along with human growth hormone and adrenal corticotrophin (ACTH).

Thymosin is a protein extracted from porcine thymus tissue. It affects the differentiation of immature bone marrow cells and the function of T-lymphocytes.

This thymic hormone stimulates killer cell lymphocyte activity in the spleen cell cultures obtained from old mice. The serum level of Thymulin decreases with age, and it coincides with thymus atrophy. Thymulin requires zinc for full biological activity.

Patients who suffer from Crohn's disease or acute lymphoblastic leukemia are Zinc deficient. They also have a reduction in Thymulin activity. Young and old rats increased circulating Thymulin levels in response to administration of growth hormone and thyroid hormone injections.

THF is an extract of calf thymus. Interleukin-2 is a protein manufactured by lymphocytes. It was enhanced by the influence of THF in spleen cell cultures. Peripheral blood obtained from patients with chronic hepatitis B and viral infections responded to THF with increased production of IL-2. This suggests a possible antiviral role for this thymic hormone.

Thymopoietin is a protein isolated from bovine thymus gland. Thymopoietin enhances T-lymphocyte differentiation and effect of function on mature T-lymphocytes.

Various studies teach that the thymus gland and thymic hormones contribute to human immunity and to the neuroendocrine system. Additionally, alteration in the status of the thyroid, adrenal, and pituitary glands, as well as the kidney, have affected the structure and function of the thymus gland. Finally, results indicate that the presence of thymic hormone in circulation can have an affect on a variety of other organ systems.

Studies and tests have thus shown that thymus hormone replacement therapy tends to revitalize the body and contribute to more youthful performance of our various systems:

Immune

Neuroendocrine

Reproductive

Central nervous

In summary, replacement of thymic hormone elements greatly enhances the immune system and tends to inhibit many age-related diseases.

2) Adverse Side Effects of Thymic HRT

There have been no adverse side effects noted.

Chapter 4.9 Thyroid Hormone

Thyroid hormone (TH) is the principle hormone that regulates our production of energy, metabolism, temperature, and heart rate. It must be available in its optimum amount for us to have optimum health.

Thyroid hormones are the source of our vitality and youth.

Thyroid hormone is secreted by the thyroid gland that is positioned in the base of the neck. It regulates our metabolism by controlling the production of energy in our cells. The fuel from food and stored fat combines with oxygen in our cells to produce the chemical energy that powers all the functions of our body from movement to thought. The thyroid hormone, thyroxin, is the regulator of this process and the controller of our body heat and rate of cellular activity.

In normal, healthy people the thyroid hormone builds up with age and then, almost always, begins to decline – for most people – in late middle age. When it begins to decline with age or for some other reason, our metabolism is slowed down.

The slowing of our metabolism causes the following problems:

Fatigue and loss of energy

Weakness

Susceptible to colds and viruses

Heavier, and more labored breathing

Muscle cramps

Persistent low back pain

Bruising easily

Mental sluggishness (poor memory)

Headaches

Emotional instability

Cold hands and feet

Dry, course, leathery, or pale skin

Course hair or loss of hair

Brittle nails

Stiff joints

Reduced interest in sex

Clogged arteries

Poor circulation

If the thyroid is not secreting enough hormones, there will not be enough energy or stamina. This condition is called myxedema (hypothyroidism).

The imbalance of thyroid hormones may also be responsible for disorders such as arteriosclerosis, high blood pressure, and senility among people who are not very old.

If there is an excess secretion of thyroid hormones, as in Basedow's disease (also known as Graves' disease), there will be too much energy. The body will be quickly worn out, as the throttle is wide open for too long.

Eating too much kelp, for example, may trigger Basedow's disease because kelp contains a large amount of substances that make up thyroid hormones.

During the heavy bombing of London during World War II, an unusually high number of people in London were affected by Basedow's disease. At the onset of the Gulf War, President Bush was affected by Basedow's disease. The illness also affected Mrs. Bush and even their dog.

Basedow's disease is known as war disease because the extreme tension in the face of an enemy's attack may trigger the illness. This is another illustration of how stresses in our life can erode the balance of hormones.

Among young women, 1 in 20 to 30 is found to have an abnormality with the thyroid hormone.

Basedow's disease, Harshimoto's disease (hypothyroidism), and thyroid cancer are found more often among young women than men. Women are 5 times more likely to have abnormalities in their thyroid gland. This is because the thyroid gland and female hormones are closely related.

As an interesting side note, it is reported that among some tribes of American Indians, a bride's neck is measured to indicate how happy she is. Medically speaking, it makes sense to measure the neck for feelings of happiness or euphoria, for the neck may slightly increase in width as the thyroid responds to human feelings, swelling slightly as it produces hormones. Most of the supermodels that our young girls admire tend to be tall and thin with long, slender necks.

However, if you check the impressionist paintings of beautiful women or the Ukiyoe paintings of Japanese women, you will find women with fuller necks. It seems likely that women with high intelligence, warmth, and friendliness tend to have fuller necks because their thyroid glands are working actively.

Some people born with thyroid glands that do not function properly have been classified as mentally disabled. When given hormone supplements, many have shown remarkable progress. Their eyes become brighter, hair begins to grow, and they look more alert. This kind of treatment has gone beyond the experimental stage and is practiced clinically.

Studies have shown that more than 40% of the U.S. population is deficient in TH, and therefore they suffer from some of the symptoms listed above.

They are also more susceptible to adult-onset diabetes, Alzheimer's, memory problems, loss of concentration, and other forms of dementia. And many suffer various forms of depression and almost always are over weight. And their cholesterol and triglycerides are abnormally high.

1) Benefits of Thyroid Hormone HRT

But when TH is restored to youthful levels, these symptoms almost always cease, and many times the related diseases abate.

The Neurology Journal and The Southern Medical Journal have both reported cases in which TH supplements even reversed certain types of cancer. While there is not yet enough evidence to prove these benefits, investigations in this area are continuing.

2) Adverse Side Effects of Thyroid Hormone HRT

Too much TH will cause problems, specifically osteoporosis, and especially so in women. However, a carefully tailored dose program can insure that proper doses are not exceeded.

Chapter 4.10 Insulin

I would be remiss not to address the very important hormone, Insulin, even though I do not include it in our discussion. It is the hormone that facilitates the transport of blood sugar, glucose, into our cells for fuel. It is normally released when we eat. Some glucose gets stored in the liver and muscles as glycogen, a complex carbohydrate that the body can call upon to meet energy needs.

If insulin is not doing its job properly, then the excess glucose is more easily stored as fat and the break down of fat for energy is also impaired.

Insulin frequently becomes a hormonal problem as we get older; the body uses it less efficiently, and the resulting condition, called insulin resistance, is associated with increased obesity, high blood pressure, and cardiovascular risk. Careful diet and exercise can minimize the problem, but insulin HRT is frequently required.

Precise monitoring devices and techniques have been developed to measure glucose levels in the blood of diabetics and borderline diabetics. Generally speaking, glucose levels of less than 99 micrograms per deciliter of blood are considered normal, over 130 diabetic, and in between, borderline diabetic.

One can become diabetic as insulin resistance builds with age or when the Laggerhorn glands of the pancreas fail to produce sufficient insulin. Defective genes that cause, or allow, the immune system to attack and destroy the

Laggerhorn, usually cause the later. This form of diabetics is termed Type I or "juvenile on-set diabetics." The diabetics that start as we age is termed Type II or "adult on-set diabetics".

Either form of diabetics requires insulin HRT for survival. Insulin HRT is the second largest (after estrogen) HRT program in use today. Genetically-altered bacteria manufacture 97% of the insulin used in the U.S.A. These bacteria have had human genes that instructs for the manufacture of human insulin, spliced into their chromosomes.

I do not address the insulin and diabetics issues because detailed programs have been established, and diabetic treatments are generally well established.

Chapter 4.11 Stress Hormones

There are many other hormones that control various aspects of our daily functions. I would be remiss in not mentioning them even though I do not include them in our detailed discussions.

1) Adrenaline

Adrenaline is made by noradrenalin, and the two hormones work together like twins. Adrenaline is the hormone released instantaneously when we experience fear or danger; it is a conditional reflex.

Adrenaline prepares our body and mind for emergency actions. However, the release of adrenaline is like an explosion, and it does not last.

Adrenaline can enable us to accomplish incredible things, but it cannot maintain this ability, and its effects disappear within a few minutes.

Suppose you're walking across the street when suddenly a run-away truck comes roaring your way. You leap across the distance separating you from the sidewalk, and it misses you by inches. You notice that you are trembling, that your heart is pounding, and that your physical reaction is entirely out of proportion to the physical effort you just made. In fact, you are dealing with an adrenaline surge, which the body was able to send forth the in time it took you to save your life.

Adrenaline is simply one of the most spectacular of the body's key hormones. It provides the sudden surge of energy needed for the severe cases of stress.

This hormone evolved in our pre-human ancestors so they would have the added energy for "fight or flight." Our biggest problem with it now is that it is frequently, sometimes almost continuously, secreted because we are under our new world stresses, stresses that last hours rather than the almost instant stresses for which they were originally designed in our ancestors.

2) Other Stress Hormones

Our body's reaction to adrenaline and other so-called stress hormones and indeed to a great variety of hormones secreted by the Pituitary, hypothalamic glands, and many other secretions from localized Pituitary Hormones, and from Hypothalamic Hormones glands, are major contributors to a person's health profile.

While most HRT programs do not generally administer these hormones, it is vital that their levels be periodically monitored to properly assess the health profile of aging individuals.

Stress is one of the major causes of the rate of increased aging.

Chapter 4.12 Conclusions About Hormones

Our hormones are essential for bodily functions. However their needed levels decrease with age. Tests have shown that we can take supplements and injections (HRT) to return the decreasing levels to more youthful levels. But there can be adverse side effects.

It is safer to use precursor supplements (HPT) to provide the ingredients for the body to increase production of the needed hormone levels.

The hormone precursors described in this book are believed to be safe and effective. The FDA has approved them.

Chapter 5
Understanding Telomeres and Telomerase

"Telomeres are caps that keep the sticky ends of chromosomes from randomly clumping together; telomerase is the enzyme that adds sequences of DNA repeats to telomeres."
Walter Parks

It was back in 1961 that Dr. Hayflick determined that cells can only divide a limited number of times to replace themselves.

Then in 1982, about 21 years later, Blackburn and Szostak first presented their findings that telomeres, the DNA caps on the end of chromosomes, protect our chromosomes.

The problem with telomeres is that when cells divide to make new cells to replace aging cells, parts of the telomeres are eroded away. And when telomeres become too short the cell dies because it can no longer divide to replace itself. Then the tissue of which it is a part dies; the organ of which the tissue is a part dies; we die.

And it was back in 1984 that Greider and Blackburn identified telomerase, the enzyme that makes telomere DNA.

Our bodies manufacture telomerase to keep the telomeres sufficiently long to accommodate the rapid growth of the embryo in the mother's womb. But telomerase production significantly decreases after we are born and almost ceases as we age.

The key to anti-aging and age prevention is to re-activate the telomerase producing genes so that our telomeres can remain long enough to continue to produce new cells.

Chapter 6
Anti-Aging Treatments You Can Do Now

"The only way to keep your health is to eat what you don't want, drink what you don't like, and do what you'd rather not." Mark Twain

The best available treatments to safely prevent aging are as follows:

1. Nutracuetials to combat free radicals and Lipofuscins

2. Treat hormone decline with Hormone Precursor Treatment

3. Treat Telomere erosion with nutracuetials

4. Manage stress

5. Lifestyle, diet, and exercise treatments

Stress management, diet, exercise, and lifestyle protocols are beyond the intended scope of this book. I may address these treatments in a sequel.

Let's discuss how best to use supplements in combinations to address the first 3 simultaneously.

Nutracuetials to Combat Free Radicals, Treat Hormone Decline, and Activate Telomerase

The telomerase gene has receptors for all of the supplements described below. These receptors are also sensitive to the key hormones previously described and thereby to the hormone precursor nutracuetials also described below.

Therefore the most effective nutracuetials to activate the telomerase genes and fight free radicals are the following:

1. Astragalus Membranaceus has been designed for a 6-month program that, in tests, increased telomere length equivalent to about 9 years of extra aging.

This supplement typically re-grows about 460 base pairs of telomeres with 6 months of use.

It is noted that the following should be avoided when taking Astragalus Membranaceus:

Curcumin

Resveratrol

Quercetin

Melatonin

Green tea and cacao

Allicin (garlic)

Silymarin

The user can repeat the 6-month program on a yearly basis if so desired.

2. Resveratrol with Vitamin D3 is an annual program that, in tests, increased energy levels and feelings of well-being equivalent to over 10 years of age reversal.

It caused the cells in the body to create new mitochondria, which are the cell components that create the energy in our bodies. It also increased the blood flow to the brain and reduced the risk of Alzheimer's disease.

It was proven to be a very good fighter of inflammation. In a test with rodents it slowed their rate of aging by 92%. In a test with humans it slowed the rate of aging by 260% during the test period.

The user should not take Astragalus Membranaceus with Resveratrol.

The user can repeat the program on a yearly basis if so desired.

3. Special Multivitamins is an annual program that, in tests, reduced the loss of telomere length equivalent to 9.8 years of aging. The user can repeat the program on a yearly basis if so desired.

4. Omega 3 Fish Oil is an annual program that in an experiment with rodents, dietary enrichment with omega-3 fatty acids prolonged life span by approximately one-third.

In a 6-year study with 276 humans there was a 32% decrease in the odds of telomere shortening for those supplementing with omega 3 fish oils. This was found to be true for all ages, sexes, races/ethnicities, smokers and non-smokers, normal and type 2 diabetes, and all income and education levels.

The user can repeat the program on a yearly basis if so desired.

5. Coenzyme Q10 is the compound that gives your mitochondria the power to energize every cell in your body. This is crucial to the aging process, because when your cells and telomeres are starved of energy, they age faster.

Our body's ability to synthesize Coenzyme Q10 declines 20 percent every decade of life after the age of 21. The decline leads to deficiencies, weakness, and fatigue throughout the body. And it is estimated that the average intake of Coenzyme Q10 is only 3-5 mg per day from normal diet, which is not nearly enough to return the body to youthful levels.

In addition, many pharmaceuticals which many older people take only worsen age-related low CoQ10 levels and lead to worsened health outcomes. There are 143 known pharmaceuticals that cause decreased serum levels of Coenzyme Q10 in patients. These include beta-blockers, antidepressants, antibiotics, chemotherapy, radiation therapy, hormone replacement and, most notably statin drugs taken to lower cholesterol.

A drawback of Coenzyme Q10 is its poor absorption; therefore, only the best absorbing versions of Coenzyme Q10 should be used. Ubiquinol is eight times more powerful than ubiquinone, so you only need one-eighth as much.

Coenzyme Q10 is most effective when taken with vitamins B2, B3, B6, B12, C, and folic acid.

The user can repeat the program on a yearly basis if so desired.

6. Special Antioxidants can, in addition to their antioxidant functions, collectively also help activate the telomerase genes to produce more telomerase and thereby lengthen the telomeres and increase life span.

This antioxidant combination should include B12, Vitamin C, Vitamin A, Beta-carotene, Lycopene, Lutein, Alpha Lipoic acid, and Zinc.

The user can repeat the program on a yearly basis if so desired.

7. Pregnenolone with Carnosine is a major benefit to antiaging. Carnosine provided 15-21% improvement in telomere length in a lung study and gave a factor of 3 improvements in some other studies.

Pregnenolone has been proven to be of great benefit for arthritis, inflammation, memory, and diabetes.

The user can repeat the program on a yearly basis if so desired.

8. DHEA with Melatonin can prevent or reverse the diseases that anti-aging experts have identified as the most prominent markers of accelerated aging, including atherosclerosis (hardening and clogging of the arteries), cancer, diabetes, and reduced immunity.

Moreover, mounting evidence indicates that the level of DHEA in a person's blood is an excellent predictor not only of these age-related health problems but also of aging itself.

New research indicates that melatonin does much more than help some people sleep better. Exciting studies show that melatonin's multifaceted effects may improve treatment outcomes in cancer patients and extend their lives. Additional benefits of melatonin include guarding the nervous system against degenerative diseases, such as Alzheimer's disease and stroke, and preventing debilitating migraines.

The user can repeat the program on a yearly basis if so desired.

9. HGH Precursors tend to cause your body to increase the production of the key HGH hormone. This hormone significantly declines with age. The telomerase genes have receptors for the key hormones. Increasing your body's levels of the key hormones increases the production of telomerase and keeps your telomeres long and healthy and slows your rate of aging.

Your biological age is not the number of years you have lived but the levels of your hormones. By increasing the levels of hormones that your body can produce you can feel and function at a biological age of 10 to 20 years younger than your calendar age. A very large number of tests have shown this to be true.

The hormone precursor program is fundamentally different than the hormone replacement programs touted on the Internet and generally disapproved by the government because of its potential dangers. This program uses FDA approved nutracuetials to cause your body to produce higher levels of the critical hormones that have declined with age.

The precursors are L-Arginine, L-Ornithine, Choline, Vitamin B5, and Cysteine.

The user can repeat the program on a yearly basis if so desired.

10. Combination Program is the combination of all of the above programs, although some of the ingredients that interfere with the actions of some of the other ingredients are omitted for this combination program; specifically the following should be avoided when taking Astragalus Membranaceus:

Curcumin

Resveratrol

Quercetin

Melatonin

Green tea and cacao

Allicin (garlic)

Silymarin

This protocol is the most that you can do to slow aging without resorting to some of the Internet-touted programs that are considered to be too dangerous.

The user can repeat the program on a yearly basis if so desired.

Summary: This total program consists of 13 daily pills with 7 taken in the AM and 6 taken at night.

I have purposefully omitted dose levels because you should get these from your doctor. You should not use any Age Prevention Program unless you are under the care of your doctor.

Chapter 7

Test Results and Measurements

"Beauty is in the eye of the beholder and it may be necessary from time to time to give a stupid or misinformed beholder a black eye." Miss Piggy

So we know what causes aging and how we may slow it and thereby live long enough to be available for the newer programs now in development. Some researchers believe that we will eventually be able to eliminate aging.

But how do we measure age? How do we know if we are aging as slowly as possible? How do we know if our age prevention program is working?

The most obvious measurement of age is our appearance. We can look at each other and usually give a pretty good guess of age. Grey hair, wrinkles, loose and thin skin, and extra weight are all apparent by just looking at an older person.

The easiest thing to see is weight and fat. The typical female at age 30 is 35% fat and at 80, 53%. Men are much more variable. But, as we age, almost all of us get increased fat and decreased muscle mass.

Our skin gets thinner, rougher, and less flexible. Our bones also get thinner and less dense: more fragile. Our major organs shrink, and their functions decrease.

We all become slower and feebler. Our hair gets thinner and gray. Yes, the effects of aging are visible. But, a more precise measurement of biological age can be obtained by measuring the levels of our various hormones.

Testing for the levels of several different hormones in the blood can help approximate your biological age and therefore give an indication of how well you are aging. Each of the blood elements that generally change with age can be inputted into a formula to calculate your biological age based on each of the hormones selected.

The graph below shows how three of the key hormones change with age for a male. Similar grafts can do the same for a female.

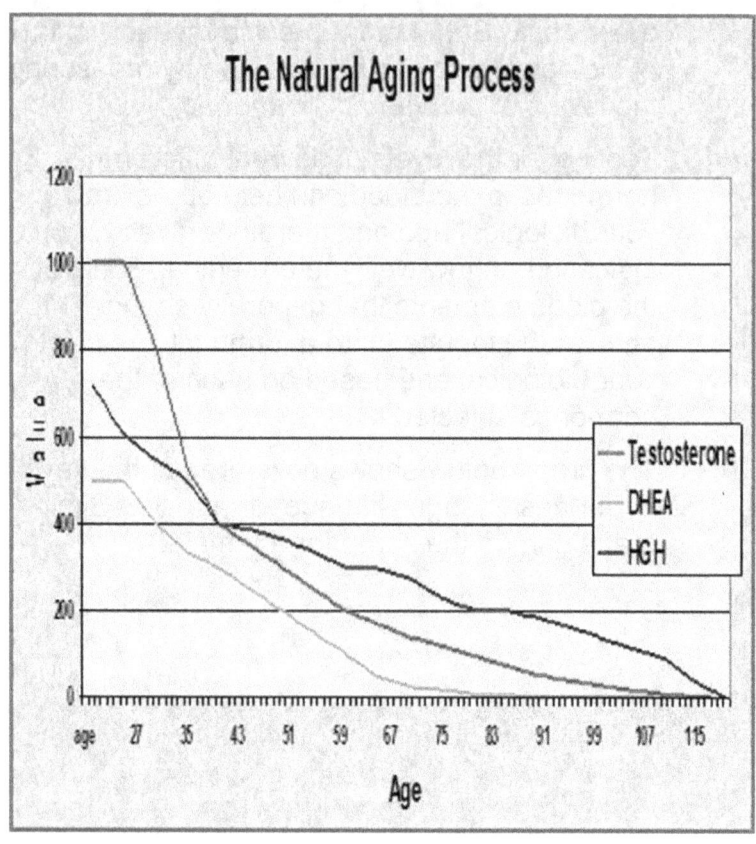

The most precise hormone measurement for age is DHEA. Blood levels of DHEA vary from person to person and average between 300 and 500 micrograms per deciliter of blood for twenty-year-olds.

The fact that some people lose less DHEA than others can explain why some people age slower than others.

By measuring DHEA, and each of the other hormones in a blood test, we can calculate one's biological age as indicated by each of the hormones.

This is accomplished by comparing your current value for each of your key hormones with the typical values of the average person. It is noted, however, that adjustments must be made for individual differences.

This following chart shows the results using DHEA as the test element for a 51-year-old man. His initial DHEA test indicated a biological age of about 5 years younger than his chronological age, suggesting that he was aging well.

However he wanted to age even slower so he took treatment. After two months his biological age, according to this one element went down to under age 27.

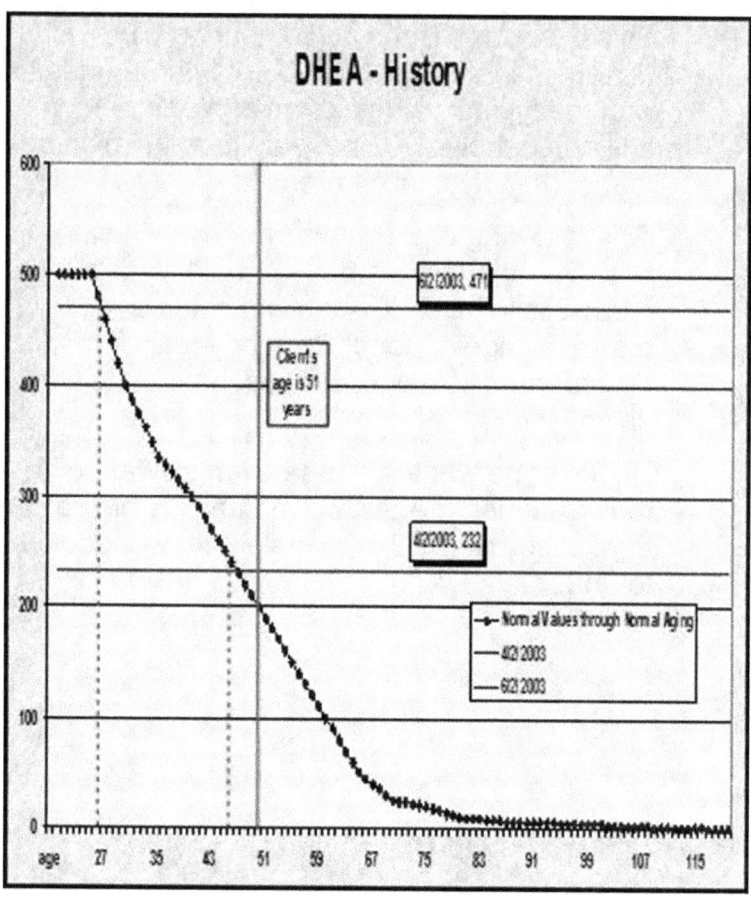

You can effectively reverse your biological age by up to 20 years by replacing your hormones to the levels you had in your more youthful days.

With such a program you can see significant results in about 6 months.

Another example is shown in the chart below for a 70-year-old man who initially had a testosterone level of 120, which suggested a biological age of about 74. He was aging faster than normal.

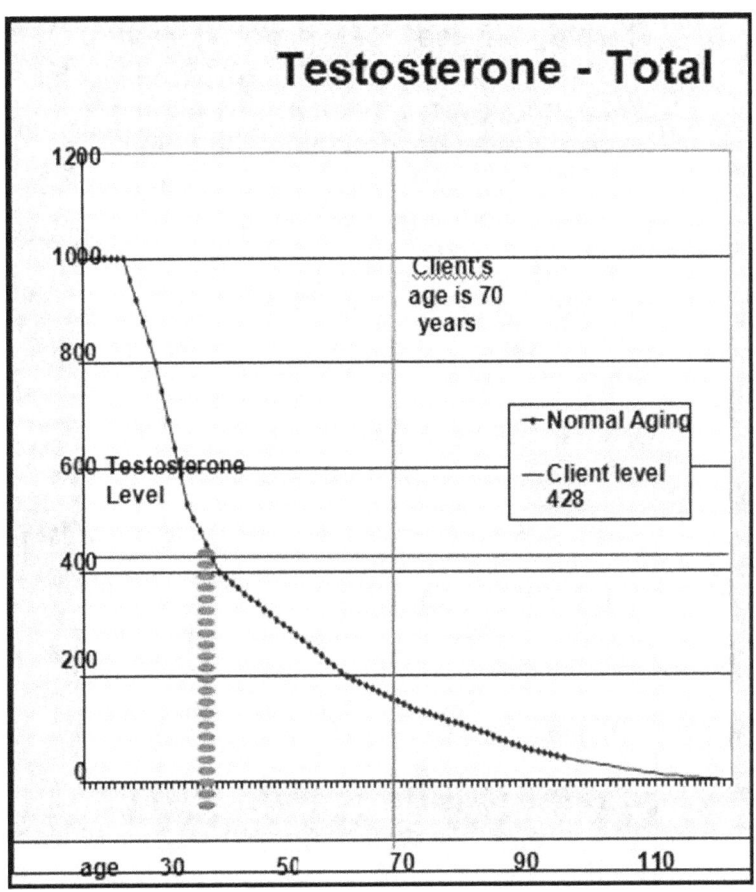

Testosterone - Total

After treatment, his testosterone level went up to 428, which indicated a biological age of less than 40.

He had been aging poorly, but treatment resulted in a very significant improvement in his biological age relative to this one element of his blood, i.e. testosterone.

Biological age can indeed be assessed, and treatments can slow down the aging process and provide a longer, higher quality lifespan.

The program used for this procedure was Hormone Replacement Therapy (HRT). HRT has been proven very effective but has basically been banned by the government because of feared risk and the potential for abuse in sports and the young.

Hormone Precursor Therapy (HPT) as described and advocated in this book uses ingredients approved by the FDA and is considered safe.

Clients taking the treatments gave their personal assessments of the tests as follows.

Fitness Benefits	Percent Benefiting
Muscle Strength	88
Muscle Size	81
Higher Energy	87
Exercise Tolerance	81
Exercise Endurance	83
Triceps Strength	61
Shoulder Strength	44
Buttocks	42
Back Flexibility	53
Muscle/Fate Ratio	25

Appearance Benefits	Percent Benefiting
Fat Loss	72
Skin Elasticity	73
Skin Texture	71
Skin Thickness	68
Sagging Cheeks	75
Wrinkled Face	71
Pouches Under Eyes	66
Skin Under Chin	63
Waist	40
Wrinkled Hands	42
New Hair Growth	38
Thicker Lips	25
Darkening of Gray Hair	10

Emotional Stability	83
Attitude	80
Emotional Stability	83
Immunity to Disease	73
Healing Capacity	71
Sexual Potency	76
Duration of Penile Erection	62
Memory	64
Nighttime Urination	57
Hot Flashes	58

HPT is not as effective as is HRT, but somewhat similar results can be approached when used over longer periods of time.

Epilogue: Search for Eternal Life

"The average man, who does not know what to do with his life, wants another one, which will last forever." Anatole France 1844 – 1924

The first immortal human may be living today.

Some scientists believe this.

Are we on the verge of learning how to live young forever? Are we realizing one of mankind's most ancient quests? Are we finding what eluded King Gilgamesh of ancient Babylon? Are we about to find Ponce de Leon's Fountain of Youth?

The causes of aging are finally being understood.

Comparatively few people are aware of the many serious scientific efforts, presently underway, aimed at understanding and intervening in the aging process, in order to one day stop aging and maybe even reverse its effects.

There are things that you can do today to help insure that you will live long enough to take advantage of the medical breakthroughs now being developed.

Discuss the information in this book with your doctor. Work with her/him to get started on your personal anti-aging longevity program now so you will be around to take advantages of all of the developing programs.

Join the race to be among the first immortals!

About the Author

Hi! Thanks so much for your interest in my books!

My principal interests are true stories of the unusual or of the previously Unknown or unexplained. I have occasionally also written some fiction.

I was born in Memphis Tennessee and grew up in Saltillo Mississippi, a small town near Tupelo Mississippi. High School life was dominated by watching the rise of our local Elvis. I was editor of the High School Paper and had plenty to write about. I guess this was the beginning of my writing career.

After graduating from Mississippi State University as an aerospace engineer I moved to Orlando Florida and worked for Lockheed Martin for 24 years. I advanced from an aerospace engineer to a Vice President of the Company and President of the Tactical Weapons Systems Division in Orlando.

<u>Education Activities</u>

I continued my education throughout my career with a MBA degree from Rollins College and with Post Graduate Studies in Astrophysics at UCLA; Laser Physics at the University of Michigan; Computer Science at the University of Miami; Gas Dynamics at MMC and Finance and Accounting at the Wharton School, University of Pennsylvania.

While at Mississippi State University I was on the President's Honor List and in the honor societies of Tau Beta Pi, Sigma Gamma Tau and Blue Key.

I received a scholarship from Delta Air Lines based on my academics and performance.

I was in ROTC and the Arnold Air Society where I participated and toured as a member of the precision Drill Team. I also attended the summer survival training at Hamilton Air Force Base in California.

I was selected for Who's Who among Students in American Universities and Colleges.

I was a speaker for several technical organizations including the American Institute of Aeronautics and Astronautics.

After Retirement from Lockheed Martin Aerospace Company

After retirement from Lockheed I formed Parks-Jaggers Aerospace Company and sold it 4 years later.

After selling my aerospace company I formed Quest Studios, Quest Entertainment and Rosebud Entertainment to make films at Universal Studios. I produced 11 films, directed

7 films and wrote 5 film scripts produced at Universal Studios.

I won the National Association of Theater Owners Show South Producer of Tomorrow Award.

I then formed UnknownTruths Publishing Company to publish true stories of the unusual or of the previously Unknown or unexplained. These include books about past events so unbelievable that most people have relegated them to "myths".

I have published 37 books in eBook format, Paperback format and Audio Books.

I have an additional 12 books in development including the following:

Walk Young describes what we can do to fight arthritis and retain and even improve our ability to walk with agility and endurance.

Remember Your Memories describes how we can retard dementia and retain our memories.

My Affair With My Heart describes my relationship with my emotional heart and my pump of life; my experiences and contrasts and heart attacks.

Ancient Memories; Genetic Memory describes the ancient memories stored in our DNA and how we can access them.

The Spring of Eternity is the story of my making the movie The Spring at Universal Studios. It is the story of Ponce de Leon's Fountain of Youth.

About
UnKnownTruths Publishing Company

UnKnownTruths Publishing Company was formed to publish true stories of the unusual or of the previously Unknown or unexplained. These stories typically provide radically different views from those that have shaped the understandings of our natural world, our religions, our science, our history, and even the foundations of our civilizations.

The Company's stories also include stories of the very important anti-aging, life-extending medical breakthroughs; stem cell therapies; genetic therapies; cloning and other emerging findings that promise to change the very meaning of life.

The Company also publishes stories from the past that are so unbelievable that they are generally considered to be myths. The published stories provide the evidence for the truth.

Please Write a Review